Oscar Pistorius.

Can a singularity throw him into jail for life?

by A. Boldireff Strzemiński

To Ewa, my wife
for thirty nine happy years we have been together.
To Ania, my only daughter
for spending so much time proof reading my work.
To Dr. Colin Sparg and his wife "Pixie"
for their valuable comments and text corrections.

Singularity explained

Is Theory of Relativity applicable to Oscar's case?

Many years ago whilst at the patent bureau in Zurich, Mr. Albert Einstein dreamt about life, space and time. Having little to do at this mundane work of his, except thinking of course, he came to the conclusion that everything in life is relative. Later he added to this thinking some mathematical formulae and in 1905 published his paper titled "Zur Elektrodynamik beweger Körper" in Annalen der Physik in which for the first time he used the term "Principle of Relativity".

Physicists say that the Universe is time/space reality and as its children made of atoms created by the Big Bang, we have to be subjects to all its laws. Hence all principles, like the Principle of Relativity, must also govern our brains and the way we act and live. There are no exclusions from such laws even though we are still unable to explain them fully, as both the Universe and our brains are largely an enigma to physicists and neurophysiologists.

Common folk cannot understand Einstein's Principle of Relativity and his "thought experiments" because they defy the logic of the world they live in. Physicists on the other hand like these experiments, because they help to discover mysteries of our Universe. But even they cannot fully explain some of those mysteries and often refer to them as singularities. This is why, even though physicists suspect that an infinitely small, hot and explosive singularity was the origin of our Universe, they still cannot describe it mathematically because infinitive singularity is non-describable.

To explain singularities better let's think about airplanes.

It should be familiar to most of us that airplanes fly due to power generated by the air moving around their wings. The wing's upper surface is much more curved than the lower, so air moves around the upper one much faster than around the lower. A physicist would say: *"velocity of the air above the wing is greater than that below"* (Kane & Sternheim; Physics, 2nd Ed. SI Version;

John Wiley & Sons, p. 282). Such unequal velocities generate much higher pressure below the wing than above. This creates an up-ward force lifting up the plane.

However, in winters, irregular lumps of ice may on occasion clog the upper surface of the wing, thus obstructing the air flow. As a result smooth movements of the air around the upper surface of the wings – called laminar flow – may change into a disorganized turbulent flow. Such turbulence gives rise to small and irregular whirlpools of air (or vortexes) which can only be seen in specially designed experiments. These may be called singularities and they could cause a plane to crash.

Singularities are unpredictable warps of the time/space reality. They may spell simple discomfort, disease, or even death. Unfortunately they may appear suddenly and out of nowhere, causing destruction not only in the papers of physicists but also in our daily lives. They often mean trouble, like singularities generated in the Atlantic Ocean, north of the equator or in the Tornado Alley in the United States, the budding source of great hurricanes and twisters respectively.

Although a part of the Universe, we live in a world created by our own brains, each one of us in an own, unique time frame. These time frames move against one another at different speeds and directions, back and forth. Reality, it seems, is not what we perceive, but what our brains build, based on strings of information received from variety of sources, external, i.e. from outside of our bodies and internal, from the inside. Often this existence becomes upset by environmental factors coming our way or due to our own actions. All such clashes with variety of factors are utterly unpredictable, hence may be seen as encounters with singularities. They throw our well organized life out of balance for a very long time, sometimes even permanently. In Oscar's life such a singularity happened on the early morning of Valentine's Day, 2013.

Oscar – a killer or a victim

Most people condemn Oscar unequivocally for different reasons. My wife Ewa, a lawyer, says: "he must be convicted and locked up for good because letting him go free may set a very bad example". The newspapers commenting on this incident also imply that he is very dangerous, quick to attack on the simplest provocation, sure of himself, always getting his way and generally unpleasant. The State Prosecutor alleges that Oscar murdered his girlfriend Reeva in rage, following a night of arguing.

This brings the following questions: How much of Oscar's true personality was Reeva aware of before they met? Did she know anything about his strange behaviour and outbursts of rage? He was a celebrity, a national hero in South Africa, a role model for school children. He was also well known abroad. She was introduced to him by a mutual friend so he would have told her how influential and wealthy Oscar was. Was she assured that Oscar could lead her into the world of celebrities, money, fame, TV and press, to be seen, photographed and to become the model, she had tried to become so many times? Did she go into this relationship for reasons other than love? If yes, we must conclude that she expected miracles but instead she paid the highest price for her inability to foresee danger: a singularity coming her way.

Many people say that love is the golden key which opens hearts and minds of people, sometimes even of wild beasts - see the You Tube story of Christian, The Lion cub bought at Harrods in the 1970-ties.

This brings us more interesting questions: Were Reeva and Oscar really in love? Openly they professed unconditional love, but a close member of her family, in an interview for an American TV Channel said: *"Reeva did not love Oscar"*. Later he added: *"the less I say the better"*. Was he telling the truth? We will never know this for sure. Adults rarely say what they really think deep inside. Usually they say what they like, depending on the situation. Only little children speak the truth because their brains are not yet fully developed. They have no memories to compare with given "live" situations. They cannot see lying as beneficial for them, until they start experiencing and accumulating this knowledge in their innate.

According to some witnesses, although already challenged by his defense lawyers during the bail hearing, Oscar and Reeva argued the whole night. Why? They were not married. They had no children and obligations they even did not live together. She came to him for this night only. Was this supposed to be a very special night turned ugly? If he was angry, why didn't she leave at the first outburst of his rage? Instead she apparently chose to stay and at about 3 am she closed herself in the toilet, two cell phones in her hands. Did she try to summon someone for help?

It is also interesting that in an interview on the British Channel 5 Reeva's mother said that they both quarrelled and fought a lot. If this is true one of explanations of this tragedy could be that they fought because they were on a verge of ending their relationship. Oscar demanded something she was not prepared to give. But at the same time she was also not prepared to drop the relationship with him so easily. An important interview had been scheduled for them a week after Valentine's Day. It would give her huge boost in the daily tabloids. Should she break away from him prematurely all her dreams and expectations would tumble down like a house of cards. She could not allow this to happen. Not just yet. She was a rising yet aging starlet on a competitive and dangerous firmament of money, beauty and modelling. Her breaking up with him would kill it all. So she stayed. Was she killed by an infuriated man unable to control his rage?

Perhaps though, there is yet another explanation of his strange behaviour. Perhaps he was not angry or raging. Perhaps he really shot her by mistake, as per his police affidavit after this tragedy.

Are all killers tried?

All mortals must die. That is why the ancient Romans coined the saying: *Memento mori*. These two simple words contain a very powerful message: remember that you are mortal. Let every second of your life be the preparation for the passage to the afterworld.

For those left behind yet another Latin maxim is in order: *"De mortuis aut nihil aut bene"*. Praise the departed or keep quiet.

This, however, creates a specific problem. How, for instance, can one praise Iosif Vissarionovich Dzhugashvili, a.k.a. Stalin, the most prolific killer in human history? Some say that Stalin probably killed close to 100 million people of different tribes and nations, even the most of his family members. (read: S.S. Montefiore "Stalin. The court of the Red Tsar." Victor Suvorov (Vladimir Bogdanovich Rezun), former Soviet GRU agent who defected to the West, wrote in his several books that Stalin designed and started WW2, the most cruel and destructive war of all times. Also, according to Suvorov, Hitler would never have risen to power without Stalin. These notions, however, are very difficult to digest, especially for the Anglo-Saxon historians, so they are suspiciously mute about Suvorov's well documented research. They hate parting with the perception of Hitler as the ultimate evil because this suits their political goals perfectly.

Biblical "a tooth for a tooth, an eye for an eye" unequivocally condemns killing; any killing. Following this advice a murderer must be hanged. Should Oscar be sentenced accordingly?

There are, however, some murderers who kill within a full majesty of law and nobody even thinks of trying them. What about politicians, who draw many nations into a war on false assumption of their imaginary enemy amassing "weapons of mass destruction"? How do we judge those that put bombs on planes to kill their political opponents? What can one say about closely related tribes fighting for the same pieces of land, committing atrocities worse than those the world experienced during WW2? What about controllers of markets who with a single stroke of a pen devaluate a currency bothering not about the economical chaos and ever increasing prices in a country they just influenced? What about pan-global cartels not contributing to the wellbeing of people? These questions cannot be easily answered because all of us, seemingly free, are in fact caught up in a web of variety dependencies from which there is no easy escape, if any at all.

So here we are: Mr. Oscar Pistorius and Miss Reeva Steenkamp. He killed her. She was a beautiful, loving and innocent human being. Was he a blood thirsty killer, raging and lustful? Was she his innocent victim? Or, perhaps, should one rather say: "it takes two to tango"? I doubt that we'll ever know the truth because she has been eternally silenced and he doesn't dare to say a thing, otherwise he might plunge himself into an even deeper abyss of great misfortune, ending behind bars for life.

As a doctor I am very interested in trying to explain Oscar's motives and behaviour from the medical point of view, so I decided to investigate it. This, after reading volumes of textbooks and articles, slowly progressed into an urge to describe my findings.

I hope they will be fascinating, especially for those who do not understand the complexity of the human brain, which rules who we really are and dictates our behaviour. I also hope that learning these facts may help readers to survive in this treacherous world, before we finally ascend into the Great Beyond without misery, but only with perpetual love.

Why we are part of the space/time continuum

Our world was born as a result of an event called the Big Bang, an explosion which created time, matter, energy and space. The reasons for this explosion that happened about 14 billion years ago in a not known region of a not known space and medium are still obscure. Literally, we know nothing about the origins of the Big Bang, or about the time just a split of a second before it, so much so that the Big Bang still remains a theory. Scientists are pretty sure however, that the whole Universe, as we see it now, started from an infinitely small singularity which for some unexplained reasons came to a being out of nowhere and exploded. Just for a fun of it.

As a result of this explosion, in an infinitely small split of a second, radiation was born, which still exists in the Universe as

Cosmic Background Radiation. This is the most ubiquitous radiation in the universe, as every cubic centimetre of the empty space of the Universe contains about 300 photons of it. This makes it about 99% of the total radiation of the Universe, the remaining 1% composing lights of all stars, visible and non-visible to us.

Further, scientists theorise that radiation of the Big Bang begun cooling immediately after the explosion and within seconds started forming atoms. At first, the simplest atoms – hydrogen – and later, by coalescence more complicated and heavier atoms arose.

The **Atom,** a name coined by Democritus, sourced from the Greek word "non-divisible", is a truly remarkable "thing". The simplest of them, Hydrogen, consists of positively charged nucleus (proton) and negatively charged electron, which runs around it. To visualize such an atom (and this is a remarkably difficult exercise for my wife who, when asked, doesn't even want to think about it) let's imagine a marble (proton), levitating in space and a pinhead sized molecule (electron) orbiting around the marble with a speed of light, at the distance of about 80 metres. Now, let's diminish this model by the factor of 10 000 000 000. This will give us a diameter of a 4.5 Ångström, which is about the proper size of an atom of hydrogen. Contemplating such a model one can realize that 99% of an atom is just a great emptiness!

If so, aren't we all empty?

However, as life has it, in every story there is always a catch and so it is with the atom of hydrogen. Physicists say it is not an electron that runs around the proton, but rather it's an energy shell caused by the lightning movement of electron around the proton, as if the electron existed in all points of its orbit, at the same time and distance from the proton. Visualizing a helicopter in flight, with a "halo" of its speeding rotor above, might one help to realize how such an energy shell could look like.

This shell is easy to calculate mathematically, but much more difficult to be envisaged or explained. It can absorb light, in other words energy, as a consequence becoming more energetic, and yet it does not flay away from the proton. It can emit light, this time loosing energy, and does not fall onto the proton either. To break strong bonds between proton and its shell/electron, one needs to apply extremely strong energy.

By all accounts, atoms should not exist at all. All theories behind their existence one can find in any textbook of physics, so I am not going to write more about it. After all I am not a physicist, just a simple medic, so what else could I add to this subject? However, the strangest characteristic of atoms needed for our further deliberation of Oscar's guilt is the fact that atoms seem to be Schizophrenic.

Schizophrenia is a disease without any apparent organic damage of the brain, popularly called personality splitting disorder. Schizophrenic patients exhibit symptoms indicating changes of the brain functions associated with emotion, reality, communication and logical thinking. They all lead to the profound alteration of the self-image and perception of surroundings. Schizophrenic people perceive their personalities as split into two or even more different beings. The well known novel, Dr. Jekyll and Mr Hide, describes it in vivid details.

So what does schizophrenia mean when applied to atoms?

Physics experiments clearly show that although atoms do exist their position and movement cannot be tested or measured. This characteristic of atoms was for the first time properly explained by the German physicist Werner Heisenberg, called ever since the Heisenberg's Uncertainty Principle.

Not touching on the complicated principles of quantum mechanics let's imagine a bullet shot out of the barrel. Using very simple technology like photo-elements, computers and slow motion cameras, we can precisely locate a moving bullet on its path. One can therefore say that in the world of "big things" or Macro around us, we can see, measure and calculate positions of all objects.

However, this is not the case in the world of Micro things.

Position and direction of movement of atoms are completely non-measurable, because in order to do it one has to shine light on them. But, as light is energy in a form of photons it may be absorbed by atoms, changing their characteristic. It follows therefore that the position of atoms or subatomic particles in space can only be calculated with a certain level of accuracy.

Stemming from the Uncertainty Principle one can theorise that each atom can exist under many different conditions and in many places at the same time. This in fact is not a fantasy as physicists can design experiments to observe consequences of an atom being in millions of places at the same time. So in essence one not only may say that atoms are schizophrenic – or by-polar – but they are "schizophrenic" to the power of millions! This allows for further hypotheses of many Universes or "many of us" existing in many places or worlds, at the same time! How can one comprehend such strange combinations?

In summary, as atoms are the most fundamental building blocks of our bodies and their characteristic cannot be properly measured and calculated and they may exist in multiple worlds, many definitions concerning our reality must be regarded as pure assumptions. This leads us to the conclusion that reality in which we live cannot be measured and expressed in any known way.

So now, questions arise: what do we really know about our world, if we, ourselves, are made up of "schizophrenic" atoms? How can we live, full of schizophrenia ourselves, perceiving schizophrenia around us? Are we allowed to judge someone else if the reality we live in seems to be only pure assumptions? These are largely rhetorical questions, but to answer them at least partly let's analyse some facts concerning the functioning of our brains.

The brain

Our brain is a truly wonderful machine, probably the best of all living things. It guides us throughout our life, days and nights, never sleeps, always ready to direct our behaviour in many ways, consciously and subconsciously. Of all our organs the brain is also the most difficult to access, let alone be quantified, qualified or cured. Knowledge of the stages of the brain's development makes it hard to agree with the Theory of Evolution, although most scientists accept it.

Common folk, though, believe that we are the Creation of God, and His best one, although judging from the behaviour of many it might not always be the case. Still more interestingly some animals, seemingly the most dangerous, may display incredible ability of love and compassion, comparable only to the best of us. (vide again: Christian, the Lion.)

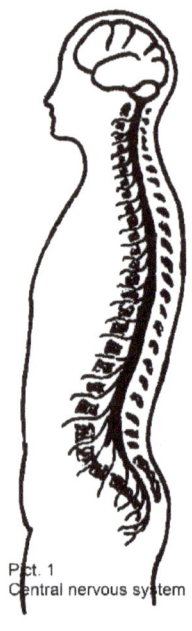

Pict. 1
Central nervous system

Anatomically the **Central Nervous System** (CNS) comprises of the **Brain** and **Spinal Cord,** which plays the following important roles in:
* Acquiring input information via sensory afferent fibres from all sensory organs (like eyes)
* Integrating received information
* Responding to this information via efferent fibres to effectory organs (like muscles)

Spinal cord is the reminder of the segmental organisation of primitive animals. This is why, together with **Afferent nerves,** which enter via posterior horns (i.e. facing the back of the body) and **Efferent nerves** which leave it from the anterior horns (i.e. facing the front of the body) retained its segmental organisation. The afferent nerves are sensory, the efferent are effectory (meaning: causing an effect). Afferent and efferent fibres unite very close to the spinal cord forming **Spinal nerves**.

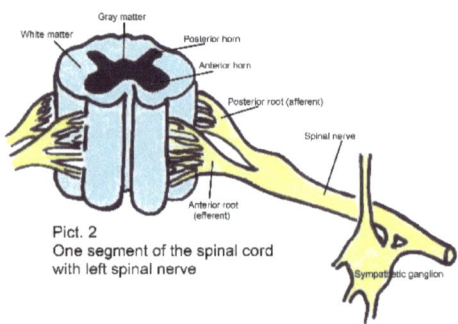

Pict. 2
One segment of the spinal cord with left spinal nerve

On each level and on both sides of the spinal cord, there is a **Sympathetic ganglion**, supplied by corresponding spinal nerves.

Spinal cord connects to the brain with a structure called the **Brain stem.** Brain stem consists of 3 parts - **Medulla oblongata**, **Pons** and **Mesencephalon**. Brain stem, which can also be found in lower animals, is the "headquarter" of important centres controlling autonomic functions of the body, among them breathing and cardiovascular. Any destruction of the brain stem, like swelling or bleeding, may quickly lead to imminent death due to cardiac and/or respiratory arrest.

Above the brain stem there are two structures: **Diencephalon** and **Telencephalon**, both jointly forming the brain's **Hemispheres**. Hemispheres developed in humans as centres of high cerebral functions, like abstract thinking, planning or problem solving.

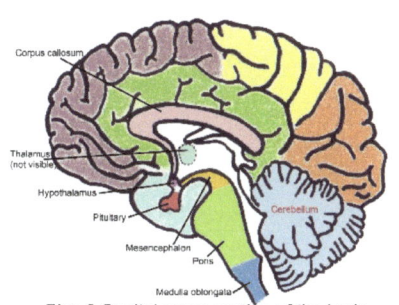
Pict. 3 Sagital cross-section of the brain

Diencephalon and Telencephalon, which are very close to one another, contain many sub-cortical grey matter centres, like:

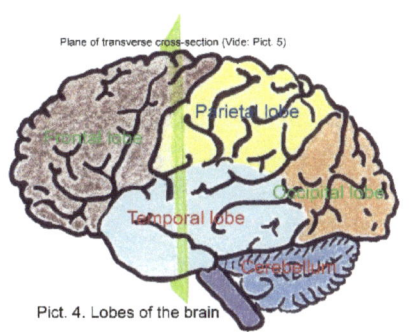
Pict. 4. Lobes of the brain

Thalamus – which controls important switching functions of sensory inputs.
Hypothalamus – which controls autonomic functions, homeostasis and integration of nervous and endocrine systems.
Caudatum, **Putamen**, **Pallidum** – which control motor functions.
Limbic system – which controls emotions; its main centres are **Amygdale bodies.**

On the outside Diencephalon and Telencephalon are covered with **Cerebral cortex**, i.e. thick layer of grey matter consisting mainly of neuron bodies. Cortex is broadly divided into four major lobes: **frontal**, **parietal**, **occipital** and **temporal**. Behind and below the brain hemispheres, at the back of the brain stem lies the **Cerebellum**, the important centre for movement control. Two brain hemispheres are connected with a structure called **Corpus Callosum** in which white fibres cross one another on their way to each respective hemisphere.

- ∞ -

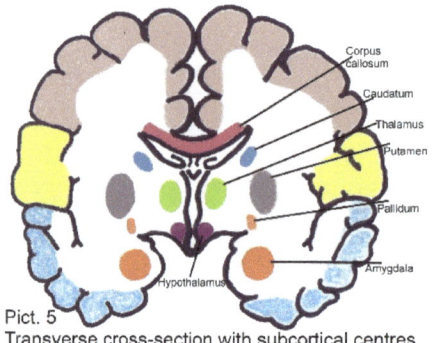

Pict. 5
Transverse cross-section with subcortical centres

All healthy humans have 23 pairs of chromosomes, all made of about 3 billion DNA base pairs, encoding for about 750 Mb of information. This is surprisingly little realising that it's about as much information as one can store on an ordinary CD.

Only a small fraction of these 3 billion DNA base pairs function as genes. The total number of human genes is still a matter of debate, but most scientists agree that we have about 20000 – 25000 haploid protein encoding genes.

Although the structure of DNA was discovered in the 1950s, and the Human Genome Project began in the 1980s, nobody is certain how many genes encode for the creation of the human brain. As this is the most complicated organ scientists agree that about 80% of our whole genome must be involved in this process. To complicate the matter further the sequence at which each gene expresses itself during encoding is even more difficult to uncover.

Our brain weighs about 1.3 kg. It is built of about 100 billion cells, called **Neurons**. Each neuron grows out several input tentacles, called **Dendrites** and only one output tentacle, called **Axon**. Axons and dendrites form exquisitely complex network of about a billiard connections, each made up of **Synapses**. In one human being this network makes pathways of about 6 million km long.

Neurons are very distinctive cells. Unlike all other cells in our bodies they resemble stars, prompting some to speculate about this obscurity. Whilst researching I found many strange ways to explain this shape, touching on mysticism, Chinese and Hindu traditions, even pictures of neuronal cortex and the Universe, which at certain unlike magnification really display close resemblance. This sounds a bit odd to me, because for the reasons of the star-like shape of neurons we must look into development of the brain which undergoes many stages, starting already *in utero* (in the womb), until finally it becomes this wonderful machine.

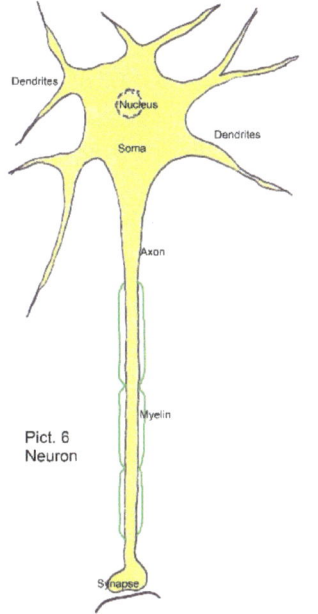

Pict. 6
Neuron

Building of the brain and spinal cord is long and complicated. The layer of the future cortex, which in adults comprises mostly of the neuronal bodies, is well defined already by the end of the first trimester of pregnancy. But these proto-neurons do not resemble stars at all. They look like ordinary cells because they have no tentacles as yet to inter-connect with one another. And only later, whilst well anchored in their positions they start budding out dendrites and axons, to connect with other neurons via **synapses,** more often than not in a far away regions of the body. Budding tentacles out of the protoplasm (soma) must pull behind some residue of the proto-neuron's interior (soma) and cellular membrane, creating this distinctive star-like appearance. This however, should not justify drawing fantastic conclusions about their resemblance to stars or galaxies.

Some nerve fibres are well insulated from one another by myelin – a type of insulation of the axon fibres which one can vaguely compare to a plastic insulation of the electric wires.

Although the inter-connecting process of all neurons starts already *in utero* it completes roughly at the age of two, under the influence of the environment. Myelination on the other hand, takes much longer to complete, for some axons it may continue even well into the third decade of life. This shows how intricate and time consuming the building of our Central Nervous System is.

Central Nervous System determines our identity and interacts with the environment. It receives information, responds to it, communicates and continuously controls acquiring all elements necessary for survival, at the same time maintaining our integrity. One can therefore say that our bodies (and bodies of other creatures, for that matter) are open/closed systems. Open, because all cells continuously absorb fresh supply of foods, water and oxygen, thereafter excreting wastes, like carbon dioxide and other products. This process, called metabolism, renews content of the cells. Closed, because metabolism upsets very rigidly kept balance of the body, so to sustain life this must be continuously readjusted to its normal level.

According to the present scientific consensus Mother Nature evolved us in a very specific way. We are descendants of simple, single-celled organisms, which originated in a primordial sea. These organisms did not have nervous systems and yet they could live, communicating with an outside world by simple osmosis, while their entire cells responded to external stimuli.

Physiologic integration

In contrast, multi-cellular organisms with their many specialised and individually functioning cells and organs could not respond uniformly to signals from the environment therefore some form of integration was required to achieve this. In mammals, evolution developed three overlapping systems of integration: **nervous, endocrine** and **neuro-endocrine.**

All three systems have senders, receivers and messengers. All of them are geared to organize responses to internal and external stimuli to meet the prime objective: maintenance of uniformity and constancy of the cells by integration of specialised responses of each individual organ. By doing this the composition of the body is maintained within narrow limits compatible with life. All three systems work during the whole life of an individual, controlling growth, maturation and reproduction.

Nervous system – is specialized for acute and quick response. It receives inputs via sensory afferent nerves (meaning: leading into nerves) and sends out information via efferent nerves (leading out), sometimes also called motor nerves.

Division of the nervous system

Nervous system is broadly divided into:

Somatic Nervous System – somatic, means bodily, serves mainly for all voluntary functions, like movements, works, daily chores; it acts via extensive network of peripheral nerves – meaning lying outside the skull and the spinal cord. They are usually mixed sensory and motor nerves containing both afferent fibres, bringing in stimuli from sensory organs and efferent fibres motorising all effectors, like skeletal muscles.

Autonomic Nervous System – controls all involuntary (or vegetative) functions. It may be compared to a computer operating system, which by using a complicated network of interactions and feedbacks, makes our bodies function perfectly without us knowing about it. In the periphery its representation consists of nerves and ganglia. An example of automatic control provided by the autonomic nervous system is breathing or heart rate. While we rest or sleep breathing and heart rate slows down; during work they automatically increase, but we don't even notice it as this is done automatically by a variety of reflexes.

Autonomic nervous system is a very important part of the Central Nervous System. In 1878-1879 Claude Bernard published papers in which he was the first to emphasize that internal consistency of the body is controlled by the autonomic nervous system.

Integrating action of the autonomic nervous system is vital for wellbeing of organisms, by regulation the activity of different organs which are not under our voluntary control. Circulation, respiration, digestion, temperature, metabolism, secretion and many other functions are regulated by this system.

The autonomic nervous system divides into a **sympathetic** and **parasympathetic** parts, both of them with opposing and contrasting actions to one another.

Parasympathetic nervous system primarily controls conservation of energy. It works during periods of minimal activity maintaining organ functions. It slows the heart rate, lowers blood pressure, stimulates the gut to absorb nutrients and empties urinary bladder and rectum. Its neurotransmitter, primarily acetylocholine, is secreted at a very slow rate, never at "full blast", thus making it rather a slow working system. It is often said that Parasympathetic nervous system is the system of satiety.

On the other hand **Sympathetic nervous system** is continuously active. Although sympathetic nervous system with **Medulla of the suprarenal gland** is not essential for survival, as de-sympathised laboratory animals can live in sheltered conditions, this system is very important during work and especially during stress. An ailing sympathetic nervous system would deprive an organism of proper compensatory reactions, like lack of vessels and heart response to haemorrhage, oxygen need, excitement, inability to raise glucose level in urgent situations like heavy work-load or stress, loss of instinctive response to danger in flight-or-fight situation and diminished resistance to fatigue. Generally, sympathetic nervous system is an extremely important protector of the organism against quickly changing stressful conditions of the environment.

Sympathetic nervous system is continuously active. Its neurotransmitters are released in small packets, but in varying concentrations at different times, depending on the need of the specific organs. Secretion of the sympathetic neurotransmitters, named catecholamines, is called **Sympathetic stimulation** and it changes continuously. At total rest the need for sympathetic stimulation decreases to about 20 % of its maximal ability for any given organism. This is the amount of sympathetic stimulation needed to maintain basic body functions supporting life like: cardiac work, circulation, ventilation, metabolism or maintaining body temperature. Decrease of sympathetic stimulation, well below this 20 % could mean loss of automatic life supporting functions which may result in death.

During stress, rage, or danger all organs of sympathetic nervous system secrete much larger or even maximum volumes of catecholamines. In such times all sympathetically innervated cells and organs of the body respond simultaneously, accelerating heart rate, raising blood pressure, compressing the spleen to add more red cells into the circulating blood, shifting blood from skin and gut into organs important for survival, like brain and skeletal muscles, raising blood glucose level, dilating bronchi and pupils, all of which as a whole prepares the organism for **flight-or-fight**.

Many other hormones and neurotransmitters play an important role in rage, under the control of **Hypothalamus**, which receives signals from almost all possible sources in the central nervous system. Therefore hypothalamus is one of the most important "relay" centres in our brain. It collects information concerning the well-being of the body, which in turn is used to control the secretion of many globally important hormones. A very important gland, the **Pituitary**, is under continuous influence, hormonal and neuronal, from hypothalamus, regulating levels of many hormones necessary to sustain the development and life of an organism.

The Synapse

Each **Synapse** consists of a **presynaptic plate, synaptic cleft** and **postsynaptic plate**, with **receptors**. When electric impulse travels down the axon and reaches the presynaptic plate a certain amount of the **Neurotransmitter** (specific to a given axon) is released into the synaptic cleft. Upon their release molecules of neurotransmitter cross synaptic cleft, reach receptors in the postsynaptic plate and stimulate them. This evokes an electric impulse (**action potential**) which travels further in the postsynaptic nerve. Essentially one may call synapses a biological equivalent of electronic diodes which force one-way movement of the electric impulses along the nervous pathways.

This concept of electric impulses along the nervous pathways must be however clarified. It is not a current of electrons, like in electric wires. It is rather an influx and efflux of different, electrically charged ions (Na^+, K^+, Cl^-, etc.) in and out of the neurons, called electric impulses just for simplicity.

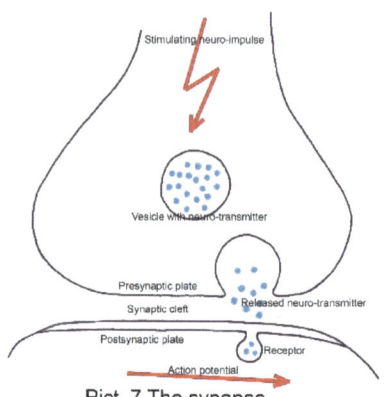

Pict. 7 The synapse

Synapses may appear on any neuron, axon or dendrite, connecting different nerve fibres together. Due to the complexity and intricacy of the neuronal net electric impulses, originating in any given part of the central or peripheral nervous system may be amplified, damped, inhibited, circulating in this region or be completely erased. Short-lived memory, for instance, is nothing else but electric currents circulating along several nerves and synapses in a given region of cortex. However, if these currents circulate in the same region for a long time they may produce changes to the structure and functioning of the proteins of this region. This results in formation of long term memory. The ancient Romans knew this already by saying: *Repetitio est mater studiorum*, meaning: repeating or uttering the same phrases over and over again makes one learn and remember.

According to the **Hebbian** theory process of learning is time related. Repeatedly active several neurons connect together so that activity of one of them facilitates activity of all others. This enlarges already existing synapses, possibly forming new synaptic connections or even hypothetical **engrams**.

An interesting fact concerning learning is **Synaptic plasticity**, i.e. a change of synaptic activity. Synapses may change their strength of response due to use or disuse, due to alteration of number of receptors, due to quality and quantity of neurotransmitters or externally administered drugs. It is now accepted that synaptic plasticity plays a crucial role in the process of learning and building up long time memory.

Endocrine system (hormonal) – is specialized for prolonged and chronic responses. Broadly, it consists of two components:

1. **peripheral glands** of endocrine secretion i.e. specialized group of cells, forming one organ which secrete molecules they produce straight into the blood stream. Best example of such an organ is the thyroid gland.

2. **specialised endocrine cells**, distributed among tissues and organs of non-endocrine functions, also secrete their produce directly into the blood stream. Hormone producing **Islet of Langerhans**, dispersed within pancreatic tissue, are their best example.

Endocrine system controls nutrition, growth, internal homeostasis and reproduction. It receives signals from the extra-cellular fluid and their messengers are hormones, both water and lipid soluble.

Endocrine system is important as not all cells of the body can be controlled directly by nerves. On the other hand, released into the blood stream, hormones have ability to reach all cells, but excite those having specialised receptors on their membranes. Endocrine system is also under the control of the Central Nervous System so indirectly CNS has a potential to influence all cells of the body.

Neuro-endocrine system – it combines both, nervous and endocrine systems, with ability of converting the electric signals received from stimulated nerve endings into chemical signals. This happens when electric signals transmitted via nerves, upon reaching certain cells or organs stimulate them for production of specific neurotransmitters or hormones, released into the blood stream.

Hypothalamus, a part of Diencephalon, is the principal structure of the neuro-endocrine system responsible for homeostatic control. Hypothalamus receives signals from almost all regions of the brain as well as from **Thalamus.** Further, Hypothalamus stimulates **Pituitary gland**, which in turn secretes variety of tropic hormones and hormone controlling factors (RF&IF). Pituitary gland is under continuous feedback control to maintain proper concentration of all hormones in the body.

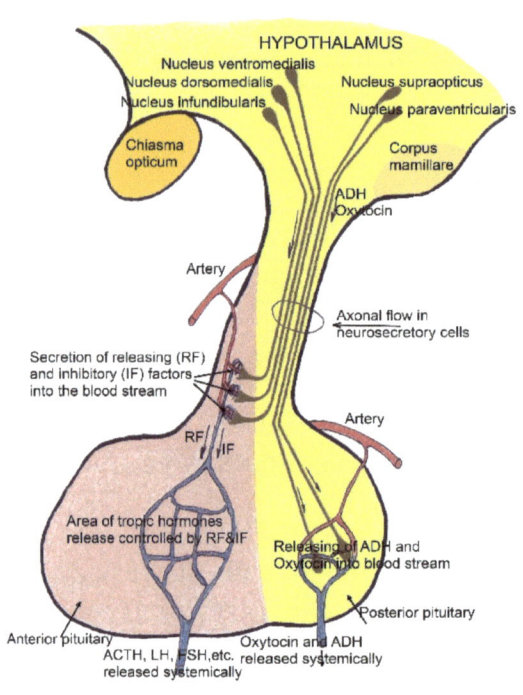

Pict. 8 Hypothalamus and Pituitary gland

Hypothalamus integrates sensory, motor, autonomic and endocrine functions, responding to continuous changes taking place in the body. It controls blood pressure, temperature, thirst, nutrition, reproduction, endocrine and autonomic activity of the body. It also prepares organism for **flight-or-fight** reaction.

There are two groups of neuronal cells located in hypothalamus:

1. **large-neurons group of cells** (supra-opticus and para-ventricularis nuclei) axons of which reach the **posterior part of the pituitary gland**. These cells produce **Oxytocin** and **Anti-Diuretic Hormone** (ADH), which by the **Axonal flow** go to the **posterior pituitary,** to be later released into the systemic circulation. Oxytocin and ADH act on uterus, breasts and kidneys.

2. **small-neurons group of cells** (ventro-medialis, dorso-medialis, infundibularis nuclei) producing variety of **RF** (releasing factors) and **IF** (inhibitory factors), each one of them controlling the levels of their specific hormones. All factors, also by **Axonal**

flow go down to the **anterior pituitary**. Both types of factors, released into the micro-circulation of the **anterior pituitary gland,** act on the cells there, controlling production and secretion of the whole spectrum of **tropic hormones** in the precise feed-backed fashion. These tropic hormones (like ACTH, FSH, LH, TSH etc.) released into the systemic circulation of the body act further on their specific target peripheral endocrine glands.

There is however, an additional overlapping of both systems in **Adrenal Medulla** and **Pineal Body**.

Defense of the organism

All three systems serve one of the most important functions of the organism – **defense against changes in the environment**, helping the organism to survive. Defense broadly consists of three responses: **homeostasis, immunity and stress.**

Homeostasis means maintenance of a constant steady state of the body. Organism must maintain constant temperature, concentration of all elements, hormones and all molecules which make up the building blocks of our bodies. But it must also get some molecules from the environment, like food and oxygen and excrete products of metabolism. Without homeostasis all these processes would quickly fail.

Homeostatic mechanism has several characteristics:
* it allows organism to check, control and detect its normal contents;
* it allows input of nutrients and output of metabolites;
* it allows process of adjusting gain or loss and signalling both of them;
* it restores system to the original level in case changes occur.

Simple example of homeostasis is maintaining constant temperature of the body. At rest small amount of generated heat can be removed by evaporation of water present in exhaled air and by contact of the skin with the environment. But during work heat excess generated by muscles is removed by dilation of small skin vessels. This increases circulation of the blood in the skin, leading to greater sweating and evaporation which cools down the body.

Immunity – this is a process of resisting changes caused by invasion of pathogens, like bacteria or viruses. Although extremely important, immunity had no bearing on Oscar's case.

Stress – has a variety of connotations. In physiological terms it defines the response of an organism to a stimulus, but one which greatly surpasses the ability of all homeostatic mechanisms to respond to it effectively. Broadly speaking the body initiates two kinds of reactions while responding to stress: immediate group of reactions, in which many chemicals are produced and released into the circulation, like adrenaline or glucose; restorative group of reactions with longer latency and maximal effects after the emergency ends. The later group serves to restore substances consumed during the first stages of stress. If stress continues for a long time, however, it may change to a chronic one, ending up with the total breakdown of all processes, immediate and restorative, resulting in an irreversible pathology and death.

The Innate

Besides controlling all voluntary and autonomic functions which allow us to survive in a continuously changing environment our brain is also the locum of our intelligence or mind, or as the scholars say, the **Innate.**

It goes without saying that our brain would not function properly if not for the many senses we have, which deliver a true avalanche of data from the environment. It is estimated that every second of our life about **11 million different sensations reach the brain** in the form of pictures sounds, scents or touches. More than 80% of these come from our eyes. But besides voluntarily perceived sensations, like seeing or hearing, there is also a huge input from involuntary receptors. These receptors, both external and internal, inform the brain about conditions of the environment and about all autonomic functions, like breathing or cardiac activity.

To contain, systematize and not to be overloaded by all this data the brain subconsciously acts as a huge filter. It is estimated that only about **40 sensations per second** reach our awareness. For all practical purposes most of the 11 million sensations are excluded from the perception process, being probably stored as "unwanted" data somewhere in our subconscious mind. They may become dreams while we sleep.

It follows therefore that the reality we live in consists of only a miniscule percentage of all sensations delivered to the brain per second. However, due to data compilation inside the brain even these few sensations of which we are aware and regard as our true reality, we have a feeling that there are no gaps in our perception of the environment.

Every instant of our life the brain creates within itself a new picture of the outside world, by comparing "live" data from our senses with previously stored memories and experiences of our past. On this ground our brain creates a reality which we regard as our existence. This process should be understood as if the brain was a director of our vision of the world by reading the vast memories of our past and only the minute "live" fragments received from all sensory organs at any present moment. Therefore our brain forces us to see, feel or smell what it wants, as essentially all these sensations are very subjective to each one of us. If however, there is a gap in perception of "live" data from our sensory organs, the brain can easily add to this picture any required information from the vast stores of our past memorized forever in our brains.

To put it into a different perspective let's think about an electric cable with a current of a certain voltage and frequency. We want to measure this current because we can't see it directly. To do this we use a voltmeter and a frequency meter. We connect probes of both instruments to the cable and read the dials, but still we can't be certain about the correctness of the results. The instruments show us voltage and frequency, but this might not be true as all instruments are burdened with certain errors or may be programmed in a specific way.

Similarly, any direct perception of our surroundings is absolutely impossible. Only newborns can probe their external world without having their sensory input processed, compiled and compared with past experiences because they have none. They are born *Tabula Rasa*, a "blank slate", ready to be written on by the sensory inputs received from the environment. In essence it is the very environment which moulds their brains in a process depending on many factors, like the environment itself, quality and quantity of all senses and that of the brain. This moulding is completely subjective and probabilistic, specific only to a given person at any given time.

This system works so well, however, that we are convinced that our world is exactly such as we see it. This conditions us to think that all other people around us must also see, feel and touch precisely the same objects at the same time, just like us. But this is far from the truth, because in fact our senses are very limited, built and acting differently and uniquely for a given person. One could compare us to snow flakes: each snow flake is different from another. Similarly, each one of us is uniquely built, an individual in the history of humanity.

To make matters worse, each one of us is not only a unique person with unique sensory organs, but these organs are also very limited in the detection of our surroundings. For example, from among the huge spectrum of electromagnetic waves we can only see one: visible light. All other wavelengths are not detectable because we have no built-in sensors to perceive them. We can't hear ultrasounds and see infrared used by some species for navigation and communication. We cannot detect gamma rays so should a concentrated beam of this deadly radiation reach us from an exploding star close-by, we would be dead within a split of a second without even realizing it. We can't see atoms because we don't have special machinery to visualize them. A scanning tunnelling microscope can do this but still the picture on its screen is only a limited approximation of how atoms may really look.

However these limitations of our sensory organs pose no problems in our daily life. We do not need to see radioactivity or infrared radiation to survive. Only when we attempt to uncover mysteries of our Universe we have to use special tools, different frequencies or detectors. And yet, this lack of uniformity of our senses creates a very peculiar situation: of all people observing the same given event each one will perceive it completely differently.

When one sees a black cat, another person may see trouble. Someone may regard a passer-by in a dark street as a murderer, but others will scarcely notice him. This is because our reality, i.e. the creation of our brain, is a canvas on which all sensations reaching it "live" at any given time are interwoven with memories, emotions, judgements and attitudes. This huge amount of compiled information continuously hurricanes inside our brains, although invisible to others and irrespective of what we do. Looking at things, walking, talking, making something, we are constantly under the influence of the vastness of our past experiences stored in the memory and the minuteness of our presence reaching us from the sensory organs. And the longer we live the amount of experiences increase.

All "live" sensations received by our brains are analysed in the limbic system where they are compared with past knowledge in order to superimpose our feelings. The negative experiences from our past will provoke rejection of a present similarly negative situation. A positive past sensation will provoke a desire. In the end all past experiences combined with present sensations are compiled in the frontal lobes, the site of our intelligence, giving rise to our awareness, in other words a kind of a virtual feeling perceived as our reality in which we live and function day and night.

Let us now analyse the following situation:

A man attacks a woman with the intention to rape and kill her. Despite the unbearable pain she fights back, still trying to collect all information characterizing her attacker. She manages to escape and later gives this information to the police. They catch the supposed killer and in court the woman, being sure that he really was the culprit, points at him as the attacker. The man is sentenced to 20 years in prison. Only a decade later DNA testing proves that he was never even in contact with her.

What conclusions can we draw from such a scenario? It appears that more than ¾ of witnesses perceive the same event differently. They may hear voices but at different times and from different directions. The culprit can be a white or a black man. The car can be blue or green. The gun never existed. Such combinations are endless.

It happens because all witnesses have gaps and mistakes as a result of their psychic state. People "live" their reality differently from one another. Stress during a fight distorts perception. It happens continuously in extreme situations but also in our daily lives, because our brains decide about the quality and quantity of the objects surrounding us and even about the relation of these objects to one another. Theses are all creations of our brains and we are not even aware of them taking place. We think that we perceive what really exists. In fact most of our perceptions are combinations of past experiences and a small amount of present "live" input. In essence our brain can be compared to a computer creating a virtual reality allowing us to see it almost as passers-by.

Human attention is very limited although our brain forces us to think otherwise. It creates an illusion of high fidelity perception of our surroundings but rejects events it regards as useless. During one test American psychologists asked an audience to watch a football match and count the number of passes of one of the teams. Almost all gave the perfect answer, but none of the respondents noticed a man dressed as a gorilla walking across the field. This "blindness of inattention" is the result of the rejection of certain information received by our brains; otherwise they would be overloaded with junk data, unable to process the real time "live" information important for survival.

Attention, however, is very important. It may decide about life and death especially in dangerous situations. A pilot who doesn't notice another airplane flying in his direction may die together with all his passengers. A hunter, who does not see a tiger ready to attack from behind may become hunted.

Here is another scenario: someone was killed and many people saw a man running across the street, but nobody saw the actual process of killing. Police asked witnesses to describe what they saw and all of them gave different description of the culprit. This is because, observing an event we immediately compare it with past experiences stored in our memory in order to explain what had just happened. Our perception is unlike recording a movie, which can be played back later, scene after scene at will and as many times as desired. It is the process of connecting a reason to the effect especially if the reason could not be observed.

It works like this: someone was killed so there must be a killer. Killers usually run away, so the runner was a killer. This is why witnesses, even those with affected vision, would later say: "Yes, I saw him running in the street. He is the killer" although they did not see a killing. They might not even have had a good look at the supposed killer running away.

Our perceptions are mainly interpretations. Watching events of daily life passing us by, we do it incidentally, therefore negligently. We saw someone running in the street in the morning. How could we predict that a few hours later we would be examined by authorities as to what we had seen? This is why, when giving evidence, we do not describe what we really saw. Pictures of a running man cannot be read out from our memory like a playback. Even with such complicated brains as ours we cannot store unprocessed pictures as we see them unfolding, because we would quickly run out of memory. We store concepts, rather than single pictures. We can only say what we thought at the time the event was unfolding. And later, when attempting to explain what we saw in the past some facts are missing, our brains can very easily produce them, based on past experience. As normally as a running man in the vicinity of a place of murder is regarded as the suspect, witnesses would say "he run away, he is a suspect", not even knowing who the runner really was and why he was running. This is why many people end up accused of crimes they have never committed, sentenced and imprisoned for years. This is due to the fact that brains of witnesses continuously interpret perceived reality – unlike "recording it" raw – and so distort it.

We see the world not how it really looks like, but how we

interpret it and who we are. And because there are about 7 billion people on our planet there are about 7 billion interpretations, i.e. realities. These realities can be shared to a certain extend with our families, friends, colleagues at work, in this way creating a common range of the world seen. Yet we do not really know all those people with whom we interact daily that well. Even the closest members of our family might be an enigma to us. At work we react with our colleagues, but only professionally, not privately. In the street we see people once in a lifetime. We may react in unison with them for a few minutes, but quickly our ways part, so our realities split up again. But we need these pieces of common realities of our surroundings which we share with others in order to exist as a community. This reality, common and yet divided among us all, functions as an unwritten agreement of what is widely regarded as normality.

There are however, humans who think and act differently from what is commonly regarded as normal, due to different factors affecting their brains during their creation, formation and perception of their daily life. Such factors may affect their brains already *in utero* and later in life due to their destruction caused by drugs, toxins, bacteria, viruses, diseases, accidents, foods, chemicals, hormones, metabolic or psychological events which bombard our brains every second of our lives.

Drugs tend to falsify reality very strongly, as if our perfectly working "programs of our central processing unit" has been infested with viruses, like computers. LSD creates images and feelings that do not exist. Marihuana, chemically very similar to one of the neurotransmitters, has a tendency to bind to receptors responsible for the sensation of hunger. Ecstasy and heroin increase secretion of serotonin, one of the most important neurotransmitters of a healthy brain. As a result drug abusers may become hungry and/or paranoid because from a perfectly working brain, in which sensory inputs superimposed on stored memories create a world which they should normally perceive as their own, their central nervous system starts creating an unknown jungle of visions and feelings. This is why drug abusers may see different colours, insects or out of this world beings, may hear voices or even communicate with the deceased and aliens. Organic destruction of the neurons following accidents may cause very similar problems, due to breaking down of the normal pathways of neuronal electric activity. If, for instance, there is a blockade of transmission from the visual cortex to the limbic system and specifically to amygdale bodies, the centres for creation of feelings, like anger, sympathy or fear, the reality of such persons would be completely distorted.

Causes of drug dependency are so multitude that it is not possible to single out only one of them. It is popularly believed that chronic therapeutic use of certain medications such as benzodiazepines, opioids, antiepileptics and antidepressants, especially when mixed with alcohol, can lead to dependence. This must make profound changes to the functioning of the brain or even its organic destruction.

Drug abuse is a big problem of our world although in the past it was largely unknown. Graham Hancock, who himself underwent a "trip to meet his ancestors" under the shamanic guidance in South America writes in the book titled "Supernatural" that controlled use of drugs is deeply rooted in the history of mankind. He argues that to maintain health of societies and families one should go on such trips, including children, but not too often and always under strict shamanic guidance. Unfortunately, our psychologically broken or divided families, with members scattered all over the world, whose daily life more often than not mean continuous struggle to provide for basic to stay afloat, have lost the needs for such trips. Today, drug abusers are mostly people without any prospects in life. They drug themselves daily to forget about their bleak future.

In this context it is interesting to consider why all governments in the world pursue, charge and condemn drugs users, yet they allow commercial selling of alcohol and tobacco, worse still, getting a substantial return to the revenue coffers, by heavily taxing them.

I think that the answer to this question might be incredibly simple, indeed.

Abusing alcohol and tobacco causes severe pathological changes in the body, but they develop very slowly. It take decades to get liver cirrhosis, similarly, chronic obstructive airway disease in smokers builds up during a lifetime. As a result chronic abusers of alcohol and tobacco can function almost normally until retirement, all this time contributing to government coffers through taxation.

But after a successful life comes retirement. Do governments like pensioners? Rather not, the sooner they die the better. They worked their whole lives, paid taxes and all contributions, now old they are only liabilities, existing at the government's expense. They would do governments the greatest favour by dying on the very first day of their retirement.

It is however, quite a different story with serious drug abusers. They normally start "experimenting" with drugs in early youth and the destruction of their body progresses much faster than that of smokers and drinkers. Within a few years such persons become a real burden to society and the government. Barely of age and yet unable to hold steady jobs... they may produce equally useless kids... The family of a serious drug abuser must be maintained at someone else's expense, right from the beginning. And yet they contribute nothing to the government coffers...

This may sound cynical, but I think that Hancock is very right on many accounts concerning drugs. Obviously drug abuse is a problem but total prohibition won't solve it either, just like the failed alcohol prohibition in the US during the 1930s. I seriously doubt that we will ever find a way to cure drug abuse, especially now with so much global insecurity and profound economic problems gripping our world since 2008.

Destruction of the brain may start already *in utero,* while it is not yet fully developed. And here the following story comes to mind.

In the mid 1970s a 35 year old woman was discovered in England, since birth labelled as mentally retarded. However, close examination revealed that in fact she was not retarded but deaf since birth. This resulted in an abnormality of her cortical and subcortical centres normally responsible for hearing and speaking. And here is why.

Our genetic make up and the sequence of genes expression during early development of the foetus determine quality, quantity and positions of all proto-neurons of the brain and spinal cord. This process is completed *in utero,* roughly at the end of the first trimester of pregnancy. From then on the proto-neurons start building up an intricate interconnected net. Dendrites and axons, some of them very long, synapse in many regions of the body. This process is predominantly influenced by the environment.

Like the whole brain, the system responsible for hearing and speaking is very complex. It comprises of many cortical and subcortical structures allowing a child to receive and process sounds in order to recognise and understand them as voices and languages and express them as sounds or speech.

It is well known that the foetus starts hearing already *in utero*, so the humble beginning of a sound "system" must start building at a very early stage of the embryonic life. After the birth of a child this system becomes more complicated allowing for the recognition of language and for expression of speech. This process takes about 2-3 years to complete and it is absolutely essential that during these early years of the child's development both parents interact with their offspring as much as possible, instead of leaving them with nannies, aged 3 months or so, in order to return to work.

Many parents who give their professional career a priority, have no inkling whatsoever that these first years are the most important formative years in the lives of their children, as not only the environment has a decisive impact on the complexity of neuronal interconnections, tremendously influencing future intelligence of the child, but also that at the very last stage of its development the brain performs the most important operation impinging on the whole future life of a human being.

It has been discovered that after the completion of the interconnections of all cortical, cub-cortical and spinal centres a small number of neurons may still be left aside, not connected, probably due to inadequate environmental input. Although usually a few neurons are left aside, they are still alive and electrically active, sending their signals around. The brain "does not like it" because such signals are an "electric noise", a nuisance for the perfectly working neuronal net. This is why such neurons must be removed and the only "known" way for the brain to deal with this problem is by destroying them. And so, the last stage of brain development is the destruction of all "idling" neurons left aside, not interconnected into the neuronal net.

Now, let's go back to the 35 year old woman, born deaf. Due to some genetic faults her ears did not develop properly. As a result sounds, in the form of electric signals, could not reach her cortical and sub-cortical centres responsible for their recognition. This resulted in the exclusion of these centres from interconnection into the healthy neuronal net. Later, speech forming was also similarly affected. As a result, a huge number of cortical and sub-cortical neurons were completely ignored by the neuronal net and in the end, regarded by the brain as a nuisance, were subsequently completely destroyed. This left her with a brain seriously underdeveloped, so even on discovery that at birth she was not mentally retarded but deaf, no medical treatment could be offered to correct this defect.

If, however, in her early life one would have discovered her deafness offering her a cochlear implant, it could probably be possible to spare the destruction of at least some parts of her hearing centres, possibly even to teach her to speak.

The above case shows equal importance of genetic and environmental factors in the creation of a perfectly working human brain. Any faults in this process can cause irreparable damages, possibly even resulting in instability of behaviour in interacting with other people. This brings us to the following question: bearing in mind that Oscar was born with some genetic disorder of the lower legs to what extend could both these factors, genetic and environmental, also have influenced the development of his brain? Could this be the possible cause of his behavioural problems later in his adulthood?

Ideas concerning the above processes were for the first time formulated by John Locke, philosopher and physician. He wrote many papers on social issues, laying foundations of modern knowledge on which present day governments and societies function even today. Below is a short citing from Wikipedia.

****

John Locke (1632 – 1704), English philosopher and physician created the origin of modern conceptions of identity. He was the first one to oppose the Cartesian philosophy and postulated that the mind of a newly born was a blank slate (Latin: Tabula Rasa). According to him we are all born without any experience and innate ideas, and only due to the influence of the environment perceived by us with our senses this Tabula Rasa is written on. According to Locke experience determines our all knowledge slowly accumulated during our lives.

Locke also wrote that "the little and almost insensible impressions on our tender infancies have very important and lasting consequences." He argued that the "associations of ideas" that one makes when young are more important than those made later because they are the foundation of the self: they are, put differently, what first mark the tabula rasa. In his Essay, in which is introduced both of these concepts, Locke warns against, for example, letting "a foolish maid" convince a child that "goblins and sprites" are associated with the night for "darkness shall ever afterwards bring with it those frightful ideas, and they shall be so joined, that he can no more bear the one than the other."

"Associationism", as this theory would come to be called, exerted a powerful influence over eighteenth-century thought, particularly educational theory, as nearly every educational writer warned parents not to allow their children to develop negative associations. It also led to the development of psychology and other new disciplines with David Hartley's attempt to discover a biological mechanism for associationism.

****

Errors in perception, transmission and compilation of neuronal signals in the central nervous system may create a completely new and distinct world of feelings in the Innate. This may cause an unknown person to be regarded as a friend, but friends or family members as total strangers, only because images of these persons cannot be compared with those stored in the memory during the formative years.

Some cortical regions of our brains are specifically important in keeping contact of persons with their surroundings. These regions, after receiving inputs from all senses, compile "reports" of the reference to the environment and they are very often sources of disorders. In such cases the brain of a person may create an innate world completely different from that of the majority. An example: a work colleague for the first time invites you to his house. While in there he asks you to put on aluminium pants, jacket and cap, because he is convinced to be telepathically investigated by aliens. Aluminium, according to him, screens his thoughts and deeds from the aliens watching him.

Your reaction could be: he is out of his mind, not only because you know it is not possible, but also because, as a part of a bigger community of humans, you are suspicious of all behaviours which you perceive as abnormal.

However, differentiation between normality and psychological disease is not so easy. A small event may often create huge changes in our brains, resulting in the compilation of an innate world that differs entirely from what is perceived by the majority as normal. According to some estimates there are at least 80 different phobias or fears, like fear of heights, spiders or closed spaces. Some people fear events which to others are completely innocent and laughable. Yet sufferers don't see them funny at all. They still perceive their twisted reality as normal, not understanding that in fact the world in which they imprison themselves in has been created by their own mind.

About 5 % of the human population suffers from very heavy paranoia. John McAfee, creator of the programming firm, while living in Belize, was convinced of being pursed by authorities. According to his blog he sent his look-alike to Mexico in order to falsify his residence there and to leave false traces. Some speculate that his behaviour could have been caused by heavy drug abuse.

Sufferers from paranoia may think that they are controlled by others. They don't trust even their own families and very often live in total isolation. Daniel Freeman, British psychologists says: *"life is full of tangled and ambiguous experiences, for which a man looks an explanation. Paranoid thinking might be a trial to explain them".*

Changes in perception of reality may also happen to "normal" healthy people. It may be caused by a very heavy event, so strong that their mind cannot create an antidote to it. Such an event may even end up with the death of the affected persons. Simple experiments carried out by the Americans on convicts sentenced to death proved this beyond any doubts.

Here is what they did.

They took the convict to a separate room. Whilst in there they informed him that he would die from blood loss. Subsequently, they blind-folded him and cut open small veins on his fore-arm. They bled, but only in drops, too little to cause any harm and certainly not death. Than, without informing the subject they quietly pored big amount of body-warm water onto the bleeding forearm to make an impression that blood was streaming out of the convict's veins. Not seeing what was going on the subject's brain perceived it as huge blood loss, which resulted in almost instantaneous death due to neurologically initiated stress progressing into irreversible shock and heart attack.

Similar situations apparently happened in New York, where in 1938 Orson Welles created havoc by supposedly "live" transmission from a spot of an alien craft landing somewhere in the country. As a resulted several people died of heart attacks due to panic caused by the fear of the Martians.

Such examples prove that a virtual world created in our innate may not be the true reflection of the one existing around us. Our brain never sleeps. In reality or dreams it continuously allows loads of information to flow through all its structures. We cannot control this river of information at all and more importantly we can't discern reality from dreams. While dreaming the brain creates exactly the same type of images which otherwise, during day-time it would perceive as reality. This is why dreams are mostly as clear and vivid as realities. During day-time we very often go into places visited in the past, even those never seen before. Time created in an innate may stop, return into the past and forward into the future. Some neuroscientists estimate that we experience such "trips" up to 2000 times a day. Seemingly normally day-time functioning, we suddenly start thinking: "what, if I was stinking rich?" or "what am I going to do tomorrow?" or thinking about a person met a long time ago: "wouldn't it be wonderful to be married?" Time is not perceived by our brains as continuously flowing in one direction only. In certain situations it may even slow down.

David Eagleman, an American neurologist says: *"we are imprisoned in a virtual machine, our brain"* According to him our brain does not register time and reality, it creates them. He tested people making controlled but secured jumps from 50 meters high, which they thought was a real fall and found that their brains perceived time slowing down by 30 %. His explanation is that during exceptionally fearful events, amygdale bodies of tested subjects become very active while comparing present situation to all similar ones, previously experienced and saved in their memory. Such comparisons take time, more so by individuals with memories loaded with many particularly fearful events. This is why during stress each person would subjectively perceive it as prolonged, but by different lengths, although while measured with a clock, the time of the given event was equal for all the subjects.

****

The Possibilian. What a brush with death taught David Eagleman about the mysteries of time and the brain, by Burkhard Bilger April 25, 2011. Extract from an article found on internet. This article is so interesting that it should be read in full.
http://www.newyorker.com/reporting/2011/04/25/110425fa_fact_bilger#ixzz2OfxgkjyX

David Eagleman (born in 1971) An early experience of falling from a roof raised his interest in understanding the neural basis of time perception. He directs a neuroscience research laboratory at Baylor College of Medicine.

When David Eagleman was eight years old, he fell off a roof and kept on falling. Or so it seemed at the time. His family was living outside Albuquerque, in the foothills of the Sandia Mountains. There were only a few other houses around, scattered among the bunchgrass and the cholla cactus, and a new construction site was the Eagleman boys' idea of a perfect playground. David and his older brother, Joel, had ridden their dirt bikes to a half-finished adobe house about a quarter of a mile away. When they'd explored the rooms below, David scrambled up a wooden ladder to the roof. He stood there for a few minutes taking in the view—west across desert and subdivision to the city rising in the distance—then walked over the newly laid tar paper to a ledge above the living room. "It looked stiff," he told me recently. "So I stepped onto the edge of it."

His body stumbles forward as the tar paper tears free at his feet. His hands stretch toward the ledge, but it's out of reach. The brick floor floats upward—some shiny nails are scattered across it—as his body rotates weightlessly above the ground. It's a moment of absolute calm and eerie mental acuity. But the thing he remembers best is the thought that struck him in midair: this must be how Alice felt when she was tumbling down the rabbit hole.

Physically, he seems no worse for the fall. He did a belly flop on the bricks, he says, and his nose took most of the impact. "He made a one-point landing," as his father puts it. The cartilage was so badly smashed that an emergency-room surgeon had to remove it all, leaving Eagleman with a rubbery proboscis that he could bend in any direction. But it stiffened up eventually, and it's hard to tell that it was ever injured.

If Eagleman's body bears no marks of his childhood accident, his mind has been deeply imprinted by it. He is a man obsessed by time. As the head of a lab at Baylor, Eagleman has spent the past decade tracing the neural and psychological circuitry of the brain's biological clocks.

The brain is a remarkably capable chronometer for most purposes. It can track seconds, minutes, days, and weeks, set off alarms in the morning, at bedtime, on birthdays and anniversaries. Timing is so essential to our survival that it may be the most finely tuned of our senses.

Yet "brain time," as Eagleman calls it, is intrinsically subjective. "Try this exercise," he suggests in a recent essay. "Put this book down and go look in a mirror. Now move your eyes back and forth, so that you're looking at your left eye, then at your right eye, then at your left eye again. When your eyes shift from one position to the other, they take time to move and land on the other location. But here's the kicker: you never see your eyes move." There's no evidence of any gaps in your perception—no darkened stretches like bits of blank film—yet much of what you see has been edited out. Your brain has taken a complicated scene of eyes darting back and forth and recut it as a simple one: your eyes stare straight ahead. Where did the missing moments go? *(NB: Try this with a camera rolling and recording your eyes while looking into the mirror. Thereafter watch the video clip you made. You will notice your eyes moving left to right and vice versa. AB. Strzemiński)*

The question raises a fundamental issue of consciousness: how much of what we perceive exists outside of us and how much is a product of our minds? Time is a dimension like any other, fixed and defined down to its tiniest increments: millennia to microseconds, aeons to quartz oscillations. Yet the data rarely matches our reality. The rapid eye movements in the mirror, known as saccades, aren't the only things that get edited out. The jittery camera shake of everyday vision is similarly smoothed over, and our memories are often radically revised. What else are we missing?

A few years ago, Eagleman thought back on his fall from the roof and decided that it posed an interesting research question. Why does time slow down when we fear for our lives? Does the brain shift gears for a few suspended seconds and perceive the world at half speed, or is some other mechanism at work? The only way to know for sure was to re-create the situation in a controlled setting.

"Mother Nature's a tinkerer instead of an engineer," Eagleman says. "She doesn't just invent something and check it off the list. Everything is layers on layers built on top of each other, and that provides tremendous robustness." Parkinson's disease can impair our ability to time intervals of a few seconds, for instance, but leave split-second timing intact.

Just how many clocks we contain still isn't clear. The most recent neuroscience papers make the brain sound like a Victorian attic, full of odd, vaguely labelled objects ticking away in every corner. The circadian clock, which tracks the cycle of day and night, lurks in the suprachiasmatic nucleus, in the hypothalamus. The cerebellum, which governs muscle movements, may control timing on the order of a few seconds or minutes. The basal ganglia and various parts of the cortex have all been nominated as timekeepers, though there's some disagreement on the details. The standard model, proposed by the late Columbia psychologist John Gibbon in the nineteen-seventies, holds that the brain has "pacemaker" neurons that release steady pulses of neurotransmitters. More recently, at Duke, the neuroscientist Warren Meck has suggested that timing is governed by groups of neurons that oscillate at different frequencies. At U.C.L.A., Dean Buonomano believes that areas throughout the brain function as clocks, their tissue ticking with neural networks that change in predictable patterns. "Imagine a skyscraper at night," he told me. "Some people on the top floor work till midnight, while some on the lower floors may go to bed early. If you studied the patterns long enough, you could tell the time just by looking at which lights are on."

Time isn't like the other senses, Eagleman says. Sight, smell, touch, taste, and hearing are relatively easy to isolate in the brain. They have discrete functions that rarely overlap: it's hard to describe the taste of a sound, the color of a smell, or the scent of a feeling. (Unless, of course, you have synesthesia—another of Eagleman's obsessions.) But a sense of time is threaded through everything we perceive. It's there in the length of a song, the persistence of a scent, the flash of a light bulb. "There's always an impulse toward phrenology in neuroscience—toward saying, 'Here is the spot where it's happening,' " Eagleman told me. "But the interesting thing about time is that there is no spot. It's a distributed property. It's metasensory; it rides on top of all the others."

Sound travels more slowly than light, and aromas and tastes more slowly still. Even if the signals reached your brain at the same time, they would get processed at different rates. The reason that a hundred-metre dash starts with a pistol shot rather than a burst of light, Eagleman pointed out, is that the body reacts much more quickly to sound. Our ears and auditory cortex can process a signal forty milliseconds faster than our eyes and visual cortex—more than making up for the speed of light. It's another vestige, perhaps, of our days in the jungle, when we'd hear the tiger long before we'd see it.

Time and memory are so tightly intertwined that they may be impossible to tease apart." Says Eagleman. One of the seats of emotion and memory in the brain is the amygdala, he explained. When something threatens your life, this area seems to kick into overdrive, recording every last detail of the experience. The more detailed the memory, the longer the moment seems to last. "This explains why we think that time speeds up when we grow older," Eagleman said—why childhood summers seem to go on forever, while old age slips by while we're dozing. The more familiar the world becomes, the less information your brain writes down, and the more quickly time seems to pass.

"Time is this rubbery thing," Eagleman said. "It stretches out when you really turn your brain resources on, and when you say, 'Oh, I got this, everything is as expected,' it shrinks up." The best example of this is the so-called oddball effect—an optical illusion that Eagleman had shown me in his lab. It consisted of a series of simple images flashing on a computer screen. Most of the time, the same picture was repeated again and again: a plain brown shoe. But every so often a flower would appear instead. To my mind, the change was a matter of timing as well as of content: the flower would stay onscreen much longer than the shoe. But Eagleman insisted that all the pictures appeared for the same length of time. The only difference was the degree of attention that I paid to them. The shoe, by its third or fourth appearance, barely made an impression. The flower, more rare, lingered and blossomed, like those childhood summers.

✵✵✵

Modern neuroscientists say that our brain, especially the frontal lobes which are sites of our abstract thinking, creates for us an innate virtual world every second of our lives, with us in its centre, although in a sense we are rather observers of a real world passing us by. The brain "invents" different options of our interaction with the surroundings in any given situation, getting information from our senses: what if I do this or that now? Thereafter, comparing present to past examples of bad or favourable outcomes stored in the memory, the brain draws conclusions and sends signals: "do this, you will be safe" or "don't do this, it may end up in tragedy". This is a risk-free process of implementation, allowing us to predict the future by learning from past mistakes. If we didn't have this process we would make more mistakes which could cost us dearly, even death.

This is why, the more impulsive the behaviour without referencing to our past and keeping cool, the higher the possibility of making mistakes. For instance, influence of drugs, alcohol or even stress which destruct or block proper physiological neuronal processes, may lead to wrong conclusions, forcing people into situations with no escape. A good example of such behaviour is road rage, when drunk or stressed drivers may fight with one another or run away from the police causing havoc, harm and deaths.

One such road rage incident happened in the early 1980s on a fast motorway between Parys and Johannesburg, RSA. Road traffic those days was rather scarce in South Africa, with police patrols and radars almost not present, so one could drive at a "factory given" speed, i.e. at full throttle. And so, two men, both in Porches, happened to accost one another, speeding ever faster to prove which one of them was the better driver in the better car. Eventually one of them blocked the other causing "proper" response from the one feeling offended. This, obviously, was quickly answered and in no time such play turned ugly when the two gentlemen drew out revolvers and begun shooting at each other. In the end one of them died in his car while the other was pronounced dead on arrival at the local hospital.

Modern computer technology brings us ever closer to the possibility of direct interaction with our brains. Virtual computer games, especially the most advanced where players interact with

3D programme using sensors allowing them to become the centre of action, may serve this purpose. Some people object to this, however, especially if games are particularly aggressive, but according to neuroscientists the brain "does not care" much about the origins of its inputs. There are already many examples of very useful virtual games like virtual surgical theatres or flight simulators to teach young professionals their trade. Neuroscientists think that computer games are not harmful as they do not impair the perception of our brains.

As our brains create virtual innate within themselves, based on data received from our senses and memories, such input may come from any source, even from computer programmes and in some instances it may be beneficial. Virtual lab tests, in which people change to other beings, like in the movie "Avatar", allow them to overcome their phobias, improving wellbeing and mood. Although some of these tests may be useful in treating a variety of diseases others may cause fear and stress. For instance: a plank placed directly on the floor might be impossible to cross for a subject who suffers from a fear of heights, if he sees that plank through virtual spectacles, which shows it as a narrow bridge between two mountains with deep ravines on both sides.

All this suggests the following questions: will technological progress allow us one day to create our own personalities as we please? If so, how will this affect human generations to come from the legal or social point of view?

Neuroscientists say that our personality is the creation of our own brain, because all sensory inputs we receive, like visions, tastes, scents, sounds or touches are subjective, given to us by the genetic make-up from our parents and formed by the environment in which we exist from birth. All of us are entirely different beings, so our senses must also differ from one another. And so must our Innate.

The above leads us to a very interesting question. Assuming that the innate is more or less a virtual creation of our brains, meaning we can't touch and probe our surroundings directly, it is difficult to agree that one can really get a true experience of a "real" physical world outside us. This leads us to the conclusion that computer technology may allow future generations to build their societies based on entirely different standards, perhaps even resembling today's fully computerised movies. The question is: will such societies be better or happier than ours?

Flow of information within our brains

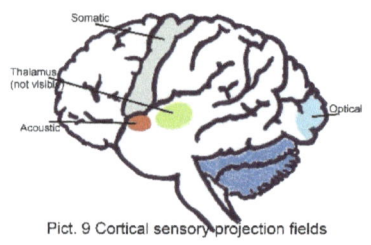

Pict. 9 Cortical sensory projection fields

Visual data, (i.e. information, input, stimuli) originating in our eyes, constitutes about 80% of all our external sensory input. There are about 125 million receptors in both our eyes, which receive pictures and convert them to electric signals, thereafter transmitting them into our brains. The remaining 20% of data comes from all other sensory organs.

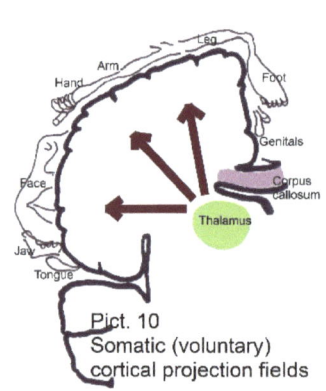

Pict. 10 Somatic (voluntary) cortical projection fields

Sensory information, converted to electric signals flow into **Thalamus**, the next important relay station which, upon receiving divides and directs them into the appropriate **Cortical Projection Fields** for further processing. There are several separate cortical projection fields for each sensory data. The biggest of them, the **Optical Cortex** is located in the occipital region. The **Acoustic Cortex** resides in the temporal regions of the brain. There are also the **Somatic Projection Fields** which integrate sensory data from our whole body, with the face being represented the most. Somatic projection fields serve as the receivers of all information concerning voluntary body functions.

Besides being a relay station the **Thalamus** also plays a very important role as a "security" organ: while we sleep it blocks some of the sensory inputs into the cortex (for instance sounds) in this way allowing us to rest peacefully.

Separate Cortical Projection Fields process all information received from the environment and combine it into logical strings,

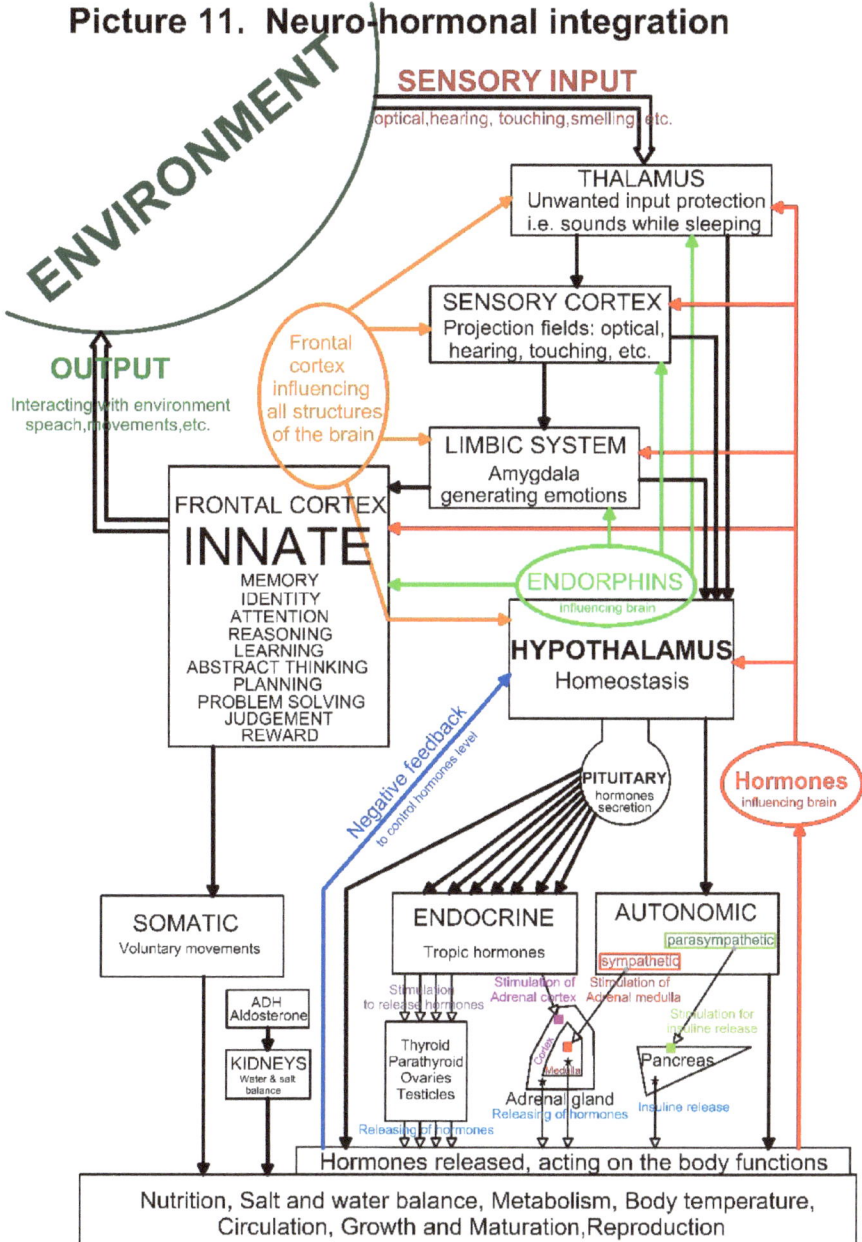

Picture 11. Neuro-hormonal integration

allowing us to respond coherently to the environmental input. This is very important as the way in which input and output are processed determines who we really are and what we are able to do. For instance: in order to learn one has to see to read a book, hear - to listen to a lecture, talk - to repeat something or to pass an oral exam. Cortex is the main centre of our awareness where all complex cerebral functions are compiled, without which our existence, daily tasks or learning and remembering would not be possible.

From the Cortical Projection Fields processed data flow further into the **Limbic system**, located deep inside our brains, where all compiled sensory inputs are further processed and exposed to emotional assessment. One of the limbic system's most important centres, **Amygdale bodies**, are the "CPU" (central processing units) of such functions, where real time "live" perceptions receive an emotional load, based on the past experience. Amygdale bodies compare "live" sensory inputs with all memories of the past stored in the brain and generate **the most basic emotions, like fear, anger** or **sympathy.** For instance, seeing a dark lone silhouette of a man in a street of a shabby suburb one immediately fears of being attacked. On the other hand, a well groomed person inclines one to be friendly. The ability to generate emotions is absolutely necessary for survival. Without them an individual would not be able to exist in the continuously changing environment.

Data from the limbic system is finally transferred into the **prefrontal lobes, the centres of our intelligence** and **abstract thinking**. These big cortical regions with neurons containing mostly dopamine receptors play the most important role in functions of the highest order like **learning**, **reward**, **motivation**, **planning, reasoning, attention, judgement** and **memory**.

Frontal lobes expose us to the surrounding world, because in order to generate proper output our innate must express itself in a logical and coherent way. For instance, a father who tells a story to his child continuously samples his frontal lobes for information concerning time when he was a child himself, at the same time communicating with his offspring by way of hearing, talking, listening and/or pacifying his spoiled brat. A teacher, lecturing pupils must continuously refer to scientific knowledge, but still, while teaching must see and react to their behaviour. A person without frontal lobes would not be able to perform such tasks.

Injuries to the frontal lobes result in profound changes of the personality. Such people cannot function properly. They display emotions inadequate to the perceived situation, for instance crying when they should laugh or vice versa, making them unable to perform the simplest daily tasks. The publicized example of damage to the frontal lobes was the case of Rosemary Kennedy, daughter of Joe Kennedy, father of JFK, the future US president. Being supposedly mentally retarded, but how exactly was never fully explained, a lobotomy was performed on her when she was 23, at the request of her father, who ordered it without informing his wife about it. In the book "The Kennedy Women" L. Leamer wrote: *"Rosemary was a woman and there was a dread fear of pregnancy, disease or disgrace"*.

Reading a short extract of the procedure performed on her found on the internet even I, a long time medical practitioner, had chills running down my spine, thinking what kind of a father could have exposed his apparently beautiful daughter to such a horrendous treatment. But knowing who Joe Kennedy really was all his life, a "skirt chaser", an alcohol smuggler during the prohibition and thanks to his riches, a hypocritical politician who, while an ambassador to the UK reported to the FDR that *"Stalin is the man to be trusted"*, after visiting him personally in the Soviet Union, I was not too surprised. It seems there are skeletons in many closets, also among the famous.

Operation called Frontal Lobotomy, developed in the beginning of the 20th century, especially the most controversial through-orbital ice-pick lobotomy, aimed at cutting off white fibrous connections of the pre-frontal cortex with the thalamus. About 20000 Americans were lobotomized in such a way and probably 20000 more in the most civilized countries like Sweden, Switzerland and Norway.

Lobotomized patients, showing severe reduction in initiative, cognition of the surroundings and detachment from society, had no ability to function without help. This resulted in much criticism with one of the psychiatrist saying: *"through lobotomy an insane person is changed into an idiot"*. As a result frontal lobotomy was banned, but only in the 1970s, partly due to the advent of modern psychotropic drugs.

After this short description of constitution and functions of the human brain we must now concentrate on its interaction with the environment as far as affect is concerned.

Affect

Psychologists theorize that during evolution *Homo sapiens* learned to display and read affect of other individuals and the surrounding environment. Affect, emotions or feelings are displayed through facial expression, gestures, body posture, words and voice characteristic. They are critical facets of interpersonal communication and vary between tribes and cultures from very discrete facial expressions to dramatic gestures and raging.

Emotions are social and psychological phenomena which occur as a result of continuous, long lasting and repeated interactions between multiple individuals and the environment in which they live. The ability to achieve their goals by each individual in a given social group depends on behaviour of others in this group and the conditions of the environment.

Emotions are complex chains of events triggered by certain stimuli. Outside observers may quantify and qualify emotions although this may be difficult because verbal communication with people experiencing emotions is far from accurate. Feelings are subjective therefore difficult to describe. People may experience a variety of feelings concomitantly, often hiding them for different reasons, so the displayed behaviour may not be an authentic reflection of the individual's actual state of mind.

Emotions are very powerful; they interfere, positively or negatively with emotions of others and their environment, changing their inter-relationships. They may affect people at whom the emotions are directed, the observers or larger social groups.

Emotions should be seen as messages which can influence the emotions, attributions and ensuing behaviours of others, therefore they may result in feedbacks directed at the causative individuals.

A good example of interaction between environment and individuals are security searches before every flight. I think that many people find them offensive, intrusive and often difficult to bear, especially when performed by arrogant security officials.

Another example are riots, like the one in London two years ago when unruly youngsters run amok in the streets, calling one another via internet to gather in specific places. One of the journalists interviewed a small group of them, their leader clad black top-to-toe including face mask and sunglasses, although it was already quite late and dark. The journalist questioned him very politely on the circumstances of his participation in rioting, causing so much misery and destruction to the community. Unabated, quite sure and visibly content with himself he replied: "because I can, and the police can do nothing about it". And indeed, luke-warm orders of the Home Minister, stemming from the, so called "policing by consent" made London police completely powerless. They could not respond accordingly while being attacked, exposing them to many injuries. Only after the prompt return of the Prime Minister, who ordered a tough stance to the violence, London streets quickly returned to normal. Does this not show that many individuals, falsely perceiving democracy as a warrant to do what they want and not getting any punishment in return push the line ever further?

The above examples clearly show that emotions of one individual evoke feelings in others, as people automatically and unconsciously tend to mimic one another's behaviour. The resulting emotion may be complementary, appropriate or complimentary to the emotions of others. Reactions to the emotions of others in a group also draw conclusions about the social status or power of the causative individual, to the result that the angry one is normally presumed to poses higher power.

Much has been written about physiological basis of emotions, their origins and variety of hormones and neurotransmitters evoking them. They are generated by the multiple structures of the brain in a complicated process in response to the external "live" stimuli perceived by the sensory organs and to the memories stored in the brain as experiences of the past.

Emotions

Although there are probably only three most basic emotions: **sympathy**, **fear**, and **anger** the possibility of classifying them is not that simple. This is because being built of milliards of the "schizophrenic" atoms we all must be "schizophrenic" to a certain degree, displaying emotion in a manner characteristic to a given person only. Each individual behaves considerably differently from one another with emotions varying in quality and quantity. To complicate the matter even further an observer of a given individual, also "an owner" of emotions, ruled by an own innate based on the past experience, must be biased to a certain degree while studying the subject. This all make possibilities of outcomes of such observations and their descriptions really staggering. And yet, for all practical purposes, psychologists try to quantify and qualify emotions into logically easily understandable groups, although some definitions are defined by themselves which adds to the confusion, making them not so easily comprehensible.

The ability of the human mind to respond to a changing environment may be broadly divided into three main ways: **cognitive**, **conative** and **affective**. The cognitive way characterizes intelligence, affective characterizes emotions and conative characterizes ability to act on the previous two. Such a definition subtly discerns meanings of "affect" and "affective", which may sound a bit convoluted.

Affect, with its many meanings, is a process in which a given organism interacts with stimulus, referring to the knowledge or skills gained by previous exposure to that very stimulus. In such a definition stimulus is a change of an environment which may or may not cause anticipated response from an organism.

Affect is closely related to experience, as the way with which an organism interacts with a stimulus may be related to the experiment, or in other words to the past exposure to the same stimulus. This in turn may lead us to concepts of learning, training and expertise. Referring to affect as experience gives us a plethora of possibilities as in our lives we are all subject to many experiences, like physical, mental, emotional, spiritual, religious, social or even virtual (via computer games) and subjective. Going further, someone with a lot of experience will be called an expert.

Affect may be **cognitive**, **conative** or **affective** and although classified as separate entities, according to some scholars all three definitions of the state of mind may at least partially superimpose on one another.

In **cognitive** affect, during process of responding to stimulus an organism employs its own mind, by reading, learning, memory, planning, or problem solving. In other words cognitive affect means processing of incoming information (a stimulus) by active analysis through the filter of past knowledge.

Conation is much more difficult to explain. It means a natural tendency or ability of doing something to get a result. This term, stemming from the Latin *conatus* (translated jointly into English words like: effort, endeavour, impulse, inclination, tendency, undertaking, striving) is somehow obscured, as it does not even appear in dictionaries of the modern English language. The closest term "con" which according to the Oxford Advanced Dictionary stems from the word "confidence" most probably does not refer to it at all. I think that if we see the word "conman" as someone with an uncanny ability to shift the minds of others into doing something beneficial only for him, we will be much closer to comprehending the Latin meaning of *conatus,* and what conation really means, i.e. how an individual with a particularly strong mind is able to twist the cognition and affection of others to the benefit of oneself.

Politicians are probably those with extremely good conative skills. They can twist and turn minds of the silent minorities all over the world the way it suits them. Here three examples come to mind although, I suppose, one can multiply them *ad infinitum.*

In the few months prior to the attack on Iraq two gentlemen, President Bush and Prime Minister Blair, managed to convince the world that President Hussein (popularly called Saddam, obviously to add further to his degradation) was accumulating weapons of mass destruction in order to single-handedly overpower our planet. Iraq was invaded, although the majority of the American and British population was probably against it, WMD turned into weapons of mass disappearance and… the two gentlemen now enjoy successful private lives, caring little about the possibility that the enormous losses of this failed war (on one stage apparently up to 1 billion US$ a day) could be the budding source of the financial crisis which hit the world hard in 2008.

Another example: on April the 10, 2010, Polish President Kaczyński and his wife, together with 94 of the highest Polish civilian, military and religious leaders died in an airplane crash near Smolensk, while on an official trip to commemorate the 70th anniversary of the Katyn massacre of 24000 Polish officers by Stalin's executioners. Not a single Western leader, like President Obama, Chancellor Merkel, or President Sarkozy honoured the state funeral of President Kaczyński and his wife with their presence. According to the official investigators the pilot caused this crash, even though in almost a hundred years of the commercial airliners' history this is the only known case when human error has been declared within a few minutes after the catastrophe and the remains of a fuselage, instead of being painstakingly rebuilt in a hangar to perform multitude tests, were deliberately destroyed. Adding to the overall confusion concerning this catastrophe National Geographic, otherwise a very careful producer of detailed air crash documentaries, concocted a slanderous homebrewed curiosity titled "Death of the President" to cover up the already well documented possibility of the explosion of two bombs on board of this plane. It seems that those with a wealth of conative skills who are the cream of world politics can deal with "insignificant" countries like Poland however they chose.

And yet another sad story: more than a quarter of a century after releasing Mr. Mandela from prison existence of the Black majority changed in an very strange but mostly unexpected way. When the politicians of post-apartheid South Africa contemplated the complete removal of the "politically incorrect" border security, installed and maintained by the hated apartheid regime, they never dreamed that it would cause an uncontrolled influx of millions of illegal immigrants from neighbouring countries, many of them infected with HIV. This resulted in spreading of this dreadful virus so quickly that more than 20% of the South African population is now HIV positive. It happened several years after the 1994 election in a country where HIV was at a very low level, contrary to all neighbouring states (read: K. Edelston, "AIDS. Countdown to doomsday"; ISBN0620129204). Total collapse of border control also caused an influx of hordes of Chinese and Vietnamese who distinctly contribute to the decimation of the biological diversity of South Africa. Killing of the rhinos for their "precious" horns that contain nothing more than cells of connective tissue are its best example.

These actions clearly show that paid politicians sitting at the "top of the food chain" use ordinary people for their own purpose as if people, borders, colour of skin or religions do not matter. This is, I suppose, because the world's majority, treated as *"nameless numbers on lists that are often mislead"*, have no say in the well controlled global mass-media.

Another way to understand the word **conation** is to see it as a faculty of the mind, desire, volition, striving, impulse – perhaps all in one, as a conscious effort to carry out acts by this mind (read: individual) who has some behavioural abilities to do them, while others have not, because their motivation is not good enough. This is why, throughout the ages, for many philosophers conation meant instigation and regulation of behaviour, *"impelling action, and by doing so it was the very essence of a man"*. At the same time, as this word has so many different shades of meaning its proper definition continues to remain illusive even for current psychologists who largely translate it to their own significance.

Here, I think, a citation is in order, which may relate to the case of Oscar and Reeva. Reitan and Wolfson have been studying brain injured patients through the lens of conation. In their paper "Conation: A Neglected Aspect of Neuropsychological Functioning" (Archives of Clinical Neuropsychology Volume 15,

Issue 5, July 2000, Pages 443-453) they explored through simple experiments how conation was affected in injured people and the capacity of the medical system to recognize how these injuries affect conation. They proposed that if the conative capacity of a person was negatively impacted, then the capacity of brain injured people to recover could be profoundly compromised, simply because they had less "drive" or "will" to heal and work through the often complex processes of recovery from brain injuries. Reitan and Wolfson continue to research this area in depth.

It could be interesting to assess the conative ability of Oscar and Reeva. Both of them had to be very persistent and stubborn by nature, especially Oscar, otherwise he would never have achieved the status of celebrity. It still remains to be seen whether Oscar's lawyers will exploit this avenue during his court case and with what an effect. If they do, however, I seriously think they should also bring Reeva into this equation, because she probably would have never liaised with Oscar if not for his celebrity status. This may indicate that Reeva was of much stronger and conative character than she ever wanted to show beyond the farce and façade of her continuously professing undying love to everything and everybody around her.

The third ability of the human mind while responding to the environment, the **affective** responses, is more basic and less problematic to assess. Many experiments prove that these are non-conscious or even sub-conscious processes, requiring minimal attention to occur, activated even without awareness. **Arousal** is one of such physiological responses to the stimulus. It is a non-conscious affective process, which may take the form of two mechanisms: one **mobilizing** and the other **immobilizing**. This process is controlled by amygdale bodies, causing the individual either to **freeze** or to **accelerate mobilization** in **flight-or-fight** reaction.

The arousal response can also be illustrated in studies analyzing the control of **food-seeking behaviour**. Earning a reward in the form of food and anticipating the reward are separate processes dissociated at the level of the amygdale bodies and functionally integrated within larger neural systems.

Mood, like emotion, is an affective state, but is not as focused as emotions. It is the set of beliefs about general expectations of future experiences of pleasure or pain and positive or negative affect. Being diffused and unfocused, mood is harder to cope with and it can last for a long time, even for years.

It is an open question whether affect is **pre-cognitive**, **post-cognitive** or even **mixed**, when initial post-cognitive events produce thoughts, evoking further pre-cognitive responses (this might be difficult to understand at first glance, so readers must repeat this phrase several times thinking about its meaning). Pre-cognition, which is questioned by mainstream scientists, means acquiring information about the future event without experiencing such an event previously. Pre-cognition touches on parapsychology, premonition, ESP events or dream-based experiences. Post-cognition means elicitation of response after some awareness process took place already, in the form of exposure to certain situations, which evoked liking or disliking experience. Some scientists also say that affect may be an instinctual reaction to stimulus, which is the dominant reaction of lower organisms.

Rage is a feeling of intense or growing anger in response to serious stressful stimulus. It may lead to flight-or-fight reaction and to violence.

Rage starts in life threatening situation and it is the chain reaction initiated by hypothalamus due to the fast release of large quantities of oxytocin, vasopressin and corticotropin-releasing hormone (CRH). This in turn stimulates the pituitary gland for production and release of large quantities of adrenocorticotropic hormone (ACTH), leading further to stimulation of the adrenal cortex for release of corticosteroids. Stress also activates **adrenal medulla** for release of catecholamines: adrenaline and noradrenaline.

Release of these hormones into the systemic circulation make profound changes in organism evoking anger with tachycardia which prepares for fast movements. It also increases blood flow to the hands preparing to strike. Increase of the adreno-medullary and adreno-cortical hormonal activity releases glucose, stored in the liver and muscles in the form of glycogen, to provide enough substrates for production of energy. Perspiration also increases, especially when anger is very intense. Characteristically, in anger noradrenaline is more strongly activated than adrenaline, but this is reversed in fear.

Scientists consider rage to be an emergency reaction, an instinct that we possess. It is a widely accepted notion that every person, when facing a threat to their pride, position, status or dignity, may exhibit some form of rage, which denotes hostile or affective aggression. According to some researchers however, rage may not necessarily cause harm to others and it is often impulsive and not planned. It is also accepted that anger normally precedes rage, but due to the complexity of human behaviour, it is almost impossible to explain adequately the reasons and conditions which make some people to continue "boiling up" from anger to rage and aggression, while others have the ability to stop and "cool down" at a certain level of anger, ending as annoyed, but not raging.

Sue Parker Hall describes anger as a positive, pure and constructive emotion that may be respectful to others, but only if it is used to protect the self on physical, emotional, intellectual and spiritual level of relationships. According to her, anger originates at ages from 18 months to 3 years, providing motivation and energy for the individual development of an innate. At this stage children begin separating themselves from the surrounding world to exist psychologically as distinct beings. During this process, parallel to the emergence of thinking, anger also builds up in such developing brains of children when something is not going on in accordance with their expectations. This is why the process of cognition may so easily arouse anger.

Parker Hall says that rage is an entirely different phenomenon than anger. According to her rage is a pre-verbal, pre-cognition, psychological defense mechanism which originates in earliest infancy as a response to the trauma experienced by the infant when the environment fails to meet its needs. It is an attempt to summon help by a terrorized infant, who feels threatened. Such an infant cannot manage emotions activated by threats which require someone else to assess and correct them. Upon receiving proper support and care infants eventually learn to process their own emotions.

Harvey describes rage as: *"a whole load of different feelings trying to get out at once"*, or as *"raw, undifferentiated emotions, that spill out when another life event which cannot be processed, no matter how trivial, puts more stress on the organism than it can bear"*.

Rage can also be caused by a traumatic event. Witnesses of the killing of a family member may start raging in an attempt to kill the murderer. Such reactions often create vicious circles ending only with death of the perpetrators or avengers, due to loss of capacity for rational thoughts and reasoning. Persons in rage may also experience tunnel vision, muffled hearing, increased heart rate and hyperventilation. They often focus only on the source of their anger. Large amounts of adrenaline and oxygen in the bloodstream of such persons may cause their extremities to shake.

Rage may influence the state of mind into believing that one is capable of doing normally impossible things. This condition is the effect of high adrenaline levels in the body which increases the physical strength and endurance level, sharpens senses and inhibits the sensation of pain. People in rage often describe unfolding events in a slow motion, probably as well as a result of high levels of adrenaline in circulating blood.

Angry persons tend to place more blame on others for their misery. This can create a vicious circle making angry individuals even angrier resulting in even more blaming of others.

People become angry when they or someone they care about has been offended, but only when:
 * they are certain about the event
 * they are certain that someone else is responsible for it
 * they feel they can still cope with it

People would be:
* angry if someone else damaged their car
* sad if forces of nature caused damage
* guilty and shameful should they personally be responsible for damage

Interestingly, people exposed to either an angry or a sad person incline to express support for the angry one. This probably originates from the fact that persons expressing anger are attributed better social status, and are perceived as stubborn, dominant and powerful. Also, people are inclined to easily give in to those who they perceive as powerful and stubborn, rather than soft and submissive.

Annoyance and rage are said to be at the opposite ends of an emotional spectrum, with mild irritation and annoyance at the low end and fury or murderous rage at the high end. Annoyance is characterized by irritation and destruction from conscious thinking. This may lead to frustration and anger. Easily annoyed people are often called irritable. Annoyance may also progress to rage, especially if it is not resolved in time and when individuals blame someone else for their misery.

Unlike human emotions **Assertiveness** was never part of our physiological make-up passed onto us by Mother Nature in the process of evolution. Assertiveness is rather a type of learned behaviour, skills of a taught communication between persons of different psychological states that otherwise cannot contact one another directly as such contacts may result in quarrels or aggression. It aims at appeasing everybody in a social group rather by appealing to the shared interests of all and focusing on an issue but not on a person. Assertiveness is distinguished from both aggression and passivity.

Assertiveness allows for a confident declaration or affirmation of a statement without the need of proof, affirming rights of all individuals involved and their points of view, without aggressively threatening, ignoring or denying their mutual rights. Assertiveness is also used to treat anxiety, its usefulness stemming from the belief that a person cannot be assertive and anxious at the same time. This is the reason why assertiveness inhibits anxiety.

Assertiveness stems from the observations that humans communicate with one another in a different manner often encroaching on each other's boundaries by questioning behaviour, opinions or needs.

There are two types of communicators

* **aggressive:** who threaten, lie, judge, break confidence, violate boundaries of others, reduce self-respect. Aggressive people do not respect the personal boundaries of others; they harm others while trying to influence them.
* **passive:** who allow the aggressive communicators to violate their rights, but later come back in order to attack the perpetrator. Passive people do not defend their own personal boundaries and thus allow aggressive people to abuse or manipulate them through fear. Passive communicators are also typically not likely to risk influencing anyone else.

In order to prevent escalation of conflict of interests into rage and aggression assertive communication focuses on issues but not on persons in this way appealing to the shared interest of all parties. Assertiveness allows aggressive and passive communicators coming to terms with one another without loosing self-respect to one another and encroaching on one another boundaries.

Assertiveness may be related to the term "agree-to-disagree", which originated about 3 centuries ago. It seems that at present this term evolved into a tactics used by inefficient and ill-educated political or administrative leaders who, unable to give right orders in complicated matters and fearing possible consequences of any wrong decision, endlessly call on so called "staff meetings". Such gatherings normally result in nothing else but meaningless disputes of a few individuals. I believe that "agree-to-disagree" creates a feeling that anything is possible. However, bearing in mind that there can only be one truth, to me this term is rather logically misleading. Let's think what could happened to an army unit should they "agree-to-disagree" to the orders of their commanding officer. This example proves that whatever we do, professionally or not, all aspects of a particular deed should be well thought out, orders should be given by only one qualified and well educated individual and their executions should be performed by well trained subordinates. Otherwise one can expect chaos, now-days plainly visible in many so called democratic countries ruled by characters whose only intention is quick self-enrichment.

Self-esteem may also predispose to rage, especially by those who have a low opinion of themselves or suffer from depression or anxiety. Such persons tend to harm others and their rage may last longer and be less focused. Such "self-inflicted" rage is a narcissistic response, caused by built up anger of past traumas, recollection of which is stored in the mind of an individual.

NB: Narcissism is generally regarded as the personality trait characterized by vanity, egoism or selfishness. Although all of us show some level of narcissism in some individuals it can reach pathologically high level. Such persons consider themselves to be the most important, have no remorse or gratitude and deny others even the least bit of empathy.

Self-esteem is very important for the wellbeing of the organism. It defines us the way we are and underlines the sense of our personal values, influencing our relation to our environment and to other people. Thus the way we think, feel, decide and act is continuously under the influence of self-esteem. According to scientists we need self-esteem as our well-being depends on self-confidence, skills, aptitude, respect and recognition from others for our successes. According to Maslow self-esteem: *"is the one which manifests in respect we deserve for others, more than renown, fame and flattery".*

Carl Rogers wrote that the origin of problems lies in the fact that many people despise themselves as unworthy to be loved. He wrote: *"Every human being, with no exception, for the mere fact to be it, is worthy of unconditional respect of everybody else; he deserves to esteem himself and to be esteemed."*

Development of self-esteem is a continuous process. It starts in childhood, continues during school years, university and young adulthood. The main factor influencing building up of self-esteem is the environment. All experiences in life of an individual have profound impact on this process; positive experiences favour development of good feelings and self-worthiness; negative ones create self-pity, lack of confidence, ambitions and respect toward oneself.

According to most scientists psychological health of a person is not possible unless the individual develops an ability to accept oneself, gaining respect from the innate self which is followed by love and respect for other persons around. This being fulfilled allows an individual to carry on with life of successes, both in family and professionally.

Self-esteem is also important in the continuous evaluation of oneself. Daily questions: who am I?; what am I doing?; is my work ok?; am I a good parent?; are important to assess and assure oneself who one would like to be. This helps to recognize innate strengths and weaknesses, allowing improvement and setting goals for further development.

Parents play a crucial role in the development of self-esteem, especially during the first few years of a child's life, showing their progeny unconditional love and the very first steps in this difficult world, teaching them to differentiate between good and bad. But even later, when a child is at school or university, the same rules apply, because academic achievements are very important sources of self-esteem. Children must be spoken to respectfully, receive appropriate attention and affection, have accomplishments recognized and mistakes or failures analyzed, acknowledged and accepted. They must also be allowed to voice their own opinions, as tests showed that children with high self-esteem had caring and supportive parents who set clear standards for them, allowing their participation in decision making while still respecting their own conclusions and views.

On the other hand, failing in life affects self-esteem greatly, as is setting too high goals or expecting children to be "perfect" at all times. Children unable to achieve these goals for whatever reasons react with stress and self-pity, as a consequence negatively impacting on their minds. One must also remember that harsh criticism, physical, sexual or emotional abuse, ignoring, ridiculing or teasing contributes to the building of a low self-esteem.

Social experiences are also important contributors to self-esteem development. While going through school or university children begin to understand and recognize differences between themselves and their classmates. Using social comparisons children assess whether they do better or worse than classmates in different activities. These comparisons play an important role in shaping a child's self-esteem and influence the positive or negative feelings they have about themselves.

Much the same rules apply in adolescence, family life or at work. Good relationships with members of the family, friends or colleagues are very important as adolescents tend to appraise themselves based on their relationships with individuals within their circles. Social acceptance increases confidence and produces high self-esteem, whereas rejection from peers and loneliness brings about self-doubts and produces low self-esteem.

People with high self-esteem act according to their own judgements, believes and principles, but they are not afraid to listen to others and accept their conclusions should they see they were wrong. They do not worry about the past, trust their own capacities but are not afraid to show their weaknesses and admit to failures. They feel equal to others but accept that there are certain variations in all of us, making each one of us unique, with special talents which should be approved. They are sensitive to the pleas of others and resist manipulation, collaboration or praying on others for personal gain.

Oscar's aggression

Since Oscar became a global celebrity he has been seen as a role model for many people, especially youngsters in South Africa.

However, after the unfortunate killing of Reeva Steenkamp this perception changed so radically that a spokesman of the South African Union of Teachers questioned recently using sportsmen as role models at all. This notion has been challenged however, with at least one scholar proposing a more docile attitude, pointing out that a role model is most of all a human being and as such, like all of us, may make mistakes.

It is difficult to say how Oscar's case will progress. Most popular tabloids around the world portray him now in a rather negative light finding ever more ugly facts from his past. They all try to convince readers that while coming of age he was a very nice and loveable boy, but getting older and exposed to fame and money he changed radically, especially concerning women with whom he became close or intimate. Many journalists described him as aggressive, citing accidents and altercations with celebrities, even with some of his closest friends.

This touches on aggression, a difficult subject, because aggression is an inseparable part of life of all higher animals and most certainly humans. It is not easy to systematize, quantify and qualify because aggression considers all aspects of our daily existence.

Much has been written about aggression in animals and humans, with many different tests proposed and researched, yet their effects are not always so clear cut, so answers are not at all that obvious.

Aggression is perceived as behaviour. It starts quite early in humans and peaks around 2-3 years of age, then on average it gradually declines, although in some children such a decline is not observed, as they fail to acquire self-regulatory ability. Such children may pose a risk to society later in their adulthood. Some findings however suggest that this is not necessarily the case and that early aggression does not always lead to aggression later, although children from the worse socio-economic backgrounds may be prone to it.

Most scientists also agree that children exposed to aggressive adults are more aggressive later in life and that corporal punishment and cruelty may deepen this even further. This suggests that child minders should interact with them in a rather quiet and tender manner. Corporal punishment is also strongly criticized for this very reason although many parents still believe that, if properly executed, it should be an inseparable part of a child's upbringing.

This reminds me of a cartoon joke I saw a long time ago. A daddy hedgehog was busy punishing his unruly child, holding him face down on his lap and hitting him with his naked hand, across the child's spiky bottom. Whilst doing this the daddy hedgehog was crying loudly and the urchin child hedgehog was laughing with content. The moral of this story, I believe, goes much deeper than this simple joke. I think that in families where members really love one another, sparsely and intelligently used corporal punishment is not considered to be a torture and probably results in more pain and aftermath to the parents than to their off-spring. It also teaches children that the ugly world of adulthood they are about to enter, may "kick them hard in the arse" should they commit stupid or crazy deeds. I therefore think that too zealous global opponents of corporal punishment, who "cry wolf" most probably due to their own miserable family lives they experienced in their youth, should not be allowed to interfere in the family lives of others. "Assume the position, Mr. Anderson" as portrayed in the movie "Dead Poet Society" should rather be considered the right thing to do.

This also brings us a very interesting question: was Oscar ever punished in a similar fashion? If not, perhaps this is also one of the reasons why he entered the world of adulthood somehow psychologically "crippled", lacking the ability to control himself in extreme situations.

There are many ways to describe aggression. Articles and books on this subject are multitude, so here is just a small extract, certainly not covering all its aspects, especially the predatory aggression in animals.

Human aggression is more difficult to define and categorize because in real life most of it happens due to mixed motives and interactions between individuals, hence it may be displayed in many different ways.

Aggression may be forceful, hostile and attacking. It may occur either in retaliation or without provocation. It may take a variety of forms: it may be physical; it may be communicated verbally or non-verbally; it may come with an intention to cause body harm, increase social dominance and manipulation, bullying or intimidation. Further, aggression may be active or passive, aimed directly or indirectly, may be related to emotions and mental states may be caused by social or non-social factors and may occur as a result of stress.

Some forms of aggression can even be sanctioned, like competing at schools, workplaces or in competitive sports. In such cases aggression plays rather a positive role, although it may easily lead to transgression from these generally acceptable limits.

Aggression may be caused by religious, moral, political, or military views and behaviour of one country toward another. In these cases it seems to be questionable, especially now when globalization allows this like never before.

In theory a united world should be better for all mankind and yet it created more divisions and prompted conditions in which big corporations, cartels, banks and the strongest countries thrive on the weaknesses of others. An example of such a country may be China, which makes up 1/5 of the world's population. Due to questionable social and working conditions China can manufacture virtually anything, selling cheap around the world, in this way destroying industries of smaller countries with weaker economies, thus leading to their social and political misery. (for example: after 1994 South African textile industry was severely compromised by the import of cheap goods from China)

On the other end of this spectrum may be united Germany, seemingly democratically ruled and of high moral standards. Its Western part, rebuilt mostly by the Americans after the post-war destruction, flourished like never before. This created extremely strong financial and industrial sector during the second half of the twentieth century. Collapse of communism, with weaker and smaller countries absorbed by the Western European economies, produced favourable condition for the united Germany to highjack control of their finances and industries. Globalization and introduction of Euro deepened this process even further, making these countries Germany's vassals and clientele.

Gender also plays a role in human aggression. According to some researchers males are physically more aggressive than females, committing the majority of murders. Males also become aggressive much quicker than females, who less likely initiate physical violence and display its indirect non-violent form like bullying, relational aggression, social rejection and mocking. Aggression can be prompted by alcohol, because it impairs judgment. Other factors promoting aggression are presence of violent objects, like guns; pain and discomfort, like high temperature (people in cars without air conditioning are prone to road rage) and frustration.

Although aggression is mostly seen in a negative light some researchers started lately questioning this traditional concept that aggression is absolutely negative, saying that intention of the aggressors is not always to harm but to increase their status. According to this view traditional researchers attribute a much stronger meaning to the most trivial forms of aggression, in this way elevating them to non-acceptable levels. I think, however, that such an attitude might be wrong considering that "zero-tolerance" to crime is now observed in many countries. Besides, in our globalised, finite and definitely overpopulated world increased status of one person has to mean loss to another or even destruction to the environment. Most probably the same applies to bigger social groups, companies, banks, cartels or countries.

Basing on animal studies one can expect that neo-cortical and sub-cortical structures play a role in aggression, the most important of them being hypothalamus and midbrain. These two structures control behavioural and autonomic components of aggression.

Hypothalamus interacts with serotonin and vasopressin, and midbrain directly connects with brainstem, amygdale bodies and prefrontal cortex, which may be responsible for inhibition of emotions, as it is known that reduced activity of the prefrontal cortex results in violent and antisocial behaviour. Vasopressin may induce male aggression and oxytocin, which regulates attachment and social recognition, may be particularly active in females by regulating bond with their offspring, in this way eliciting protective aggression.

Stress causes activation of hypothalamic-pituitary-adrenal axis which results in the release of gluco-corticoids, with cortisol being the most important of them. In humans it was found that low cortisol level reduces stress, but may result in more aggression.

Aggression is influenced by many neurotransmitters. A deficit of serotonin may cause impulsive aggression, by interacting with dopamine which is usually associated with attention, motivation and reward. Noradrenaline may influence aggression directly and indirectly via sympathetic nervous system. Another neurotransmitter, GABA although normally inhibitory, may increase aggression especially when amplified by alcohol abuse.

Of other hormones testosterone and other androgens may play some role in eliciting aggression, especially as some areas of orbito-frontal cortex may take part in impulse control and self-regulation of emotions, motivation and cognition. Elevated level of testosterone in saliva can predict possibility of aggression.

Endorphins

Endorphins mean "endogenous morphines" i.e. morphine-like acting molecules. They were discovered in the last quarter of the 20th century in the brain tissues of some animals. They are powerful bio-molecules produced in the central nervous system and function as neurotransmitters. They are complex peptides secreted in all vertebrates, during exercise, excitement, pain, consumption of spicy food, laughter, lovemaking and orgasm.

Endorphins stimulate specialized opioid receptors in the central nervous system, which play an important role in the brain and periphery modulating pain, cardiac, gastric and vascular function and possibly panic and satiety.

Opioid receptors are found in many locations of the central nervous system. Some of them, presynaptic receptors, block the release of the inhibitory neurotransmitter, gamma-amino-butyric acid (GABA), causing unblocking of the dopamine pathways, resulting in increased secretion of dopamine. The same receptors can also be stimulated by externally administered synthetic opiates, like morphine, which is not a peptide.

Dopamine, one of the catecholamines, is a very important neurotransmitter of the reward driven experiences. Each reward increases the level of dopamine in the brain. Some drugs, like amphetamine, directly stimulate dopamine receptors.

Exogenous opioids cause inappropriate dopamine release, which results in changing of the quantity and quality of the synaptic response to the neurotransmitters used by specific receptors. This may have profound effects on memory and learning (see above: synaptic plasticity)

It is still debatable which specific human activity stimulates the release of endorphins. Data concerning these processes comes mostly from animal studies, which may be different than those in humans. According to one article studies on humans often rely on plasma levels of endorphins, which may not necessarily correlate with their levels in the central nervous system. The above statement however, seems to be contradictory to the one in the following paragraph, also published in the same article. Although there is quite a lot of articles about endorphins and the blood/brain barrier I could not find definite information concerning the passage of endorphins from the brain into the blood stream.

Blood endorphins originate in the pituitary gland and placenta; brain and spinal cord endorphins originate in hypothalamus. Brain endorphins cleavage from the hormone called POMC, also a precursor of adrenocorticotropic hormone (ACTH), so levels of endorphins may correlate with that of ACTH. Blood released endorphins cannot enter the brain due to the blood/brain barrier, so only endorphins released in the central nervous system can evoke analgesia and feelings of well-being. So far there is no consensus as to the role and activity of blood-released endorphins, except for those released during pregnancy by the placenta.

The publicized effect of endorphin is the so-called "runner's high". This term refers to feelings of exhilaration supposedly due to the influence of endorphins blocking pain, perception of danger or other forms of stress. It is theorized that this process takes place in the spinal cord: when afferent painful stimuli reach the spinal cord they cause the release of endorphins which then prevent nerve cells of the spinal cord from evoking more pain signals.

Long and strenuous exercise, which ends up with difficult breathing and depletion of muscular stores of glycogen, activates secretion of endorphins. Some scientists believe that endorphins, acting in this way may even cause harm, by allowing a trainee to continue strenuous exercising despite having reached their physical body limits.

Effects of runner's high are feelings of euphoria and happiness. It has been suggested that runner's high evolved in early humanoids and helped them to survive because they hunted using method called persistence hunting. In this method hunters track their prey for miles, constantly running behind and eventually killing the completely exhausted animal. To this day small African tribes, like Khoisan, still use this method.

Khoisan, in the past plentiful peoples of Southern Africa, now almost completely extinct, used to live in small families in the Kalahari Desert. They are extremely resilient to pain and fatigue, able to run for hours and days, without stopping. Due to special habits and techniques, developed during centuries, they can survive conditions where even the most modern technology and logistics fails. Unfortunately, the last remaining Khoisan families are under threat as their homelands constitute the biggest diamond bearing areas of the world. This huge semi-desert spreading for thousands of miles from the Atlantic Ocean to the border regions of Namibia,

Botswana and South Africa is in the hands of the biggest diamond company, Anglo-American. Controlling probably up to 80% of the world's diamond market Anglo-American protect their riches, forcefully blocking entry into "their" territory in order to prohibit picking of raw diamonds which virtually lie on the surface of the desert. Those who would like to see the gone-by life-style of Khoisan should watch two beautiful South African movies "God's Must Be Crazy", part one and two.

Runner's high is nevertheless controversial due to difficulties in selecting the specific agent which evokes it. Some academics confirm it, based on PET scanner research, which compares the condition of the brain before and after exercise, although apparently other hormones, like adrenaline, dopamine, serotonin and many others may also contribute to this effect.

Endorphins are also said to be released during float tank therapy and after acupuncture, in both cases causing deep relaxation. Starting from the second trimester of pregnancy foetal placenta also secretes high volumes of endorphins into the maternal blood. This apparently plays an important role in bonding a mother with her foetus *in utero* and later while breast feeding the newborn.

Some scientists also think that endorphins play an important role in the development of **Depersonalization disorder.** Sufferers from this vast and as yet not well understood disease feel disconnected from their physical body, are not in control of their speech or movements and are detached from their own thoughts, emotions and reflections. They loose the conviction of identity and sense of automation, perceive reality as dreams, cannot relate themselves to reality and environment, have out of the body experiences, surreal episodes and panic attacks.

Depersonalization disorder is thought to be largely caused by severe traumatic lifetime events including childhood abuse, accidents, war, torture, panic attacks and bad drug experiences. It is unclear whether genetics plays a role, however there are many neuro-chemical and hormonal changes in individuals suffering from depersonalization disorder.

Conclusions

Mass-media speculate about what happened that night between Oscar and Reeva, but I lean towards two possibilities: an unresolved argument which progressed into severe rage or failed bathroom burglary according to his deposition immediately after the tragedy. This however, might not be true. He could have composed it in a hurry stricken with fear and sorrow. Nevertheless Oscar's lawyers have to stick to this line of defense, because any attempt to change it now without introducing powerful mitigating factors, may cost Oscar life long imprisonment. But before discussing this any further we must still bring to mind several important factors.

With the enormous complexity of our innate, the basic of which begins taking shape already *in utero,* it is very difficult to assess all possible deviations from the condition largely accepted as normal. This is because behaviour of anyone of us is as unique as the complexly individual neuronal make up and interconnections of all structures of our brains. To make the matter more intricate, **synapse plasticity** suggests that even fully developed adult brains may still undergo some changes when strongly influenced by the environment, so any traumatizing stimulus overcoming the ability of a given person to cope with it may utterly reshape such a person's innate.

We must also keep in mind that all cells of our bodies are under constant control of the complicated cerebral-hormonal system (vide: Picture 11). Although this system normally works very well it still has many limitations. The amount of released neurotransmitters and hormones and the number and quality of their respective receptors change continuously in accordance with a multitude of internal and external factors. This is understandable, because primarily it is a continuously changing environment that tailors our bodies to such changes while the cerebral-hormonal system protects us from this, by adapting us. One must also not forget about diseases or habits, like smoking, drinking, drug abuse or even the wrong diet, which may destroy this very delicate balance between the environment and our bodies.

Furthermore we must remember that our daily functioning, especially in difficult and stressful situations, depends on **sympathetic stimulation**, i.e. variety of catecholamines continuously secreted in small volumes practically every second of our life. They stimulate specific catecholamine receptors situated on the membranes of almost all cells of our bodies. During rest, in order to sustain the basic body functions like breathing, cardiac activity or metabolism, the secretion of catecholamines is normally about 1/5 of the maximal catecholamine-release ability for any given person. During work and/or stress it increases significantly. As catecholamines are hormones of stress one can say that we are stress-driven beings. But acting under stress is often very unpredictable.

So let's think of the following. Every day, hour, minute or even second we are slightly different persons, depending on the state of our body and mind, as influenced by the environment and as adapted to such environmental swings. One morning we may wake up in a good mood. This may fade away during a long and stressful day. Another day we feel lousy, tired, irritable. Yet another day we may be sick, with flu or throat infection and high temperature, and yet we must char at home, look after our offspring or go to work.

The point of the above divagation is this: whatever happens to us, any unusual event may strike us out of the blue when we are completely unprepared. This may result in an unexpected outcome, not only for us but also for all those around us. Besides, all of us perceive the environment completely differently from others. Therefore judging the behaviour of a "wrong-doer" by someone who has never been in that person's shoes may lead to wrong conclusions. Added to this, the legal system cannot give a definite answer to all situations we experience in real life as it is mostly based on a set of past cases and on often vaguely formulated articles that may not fit a specific problem.

We must also take into account another very important factor, already discussed. Our response to a given situation depends on the amount and quality of the memories we have stored in our innate. Looking at it differently let's think of the following: from birth we learn how to go on with our lives and discern good from bad. Learning is nothing more than acquiring models of behaviour for any given situation, at first under the guidance of parents and later under the tuition of usually older, knowledgeable professionals. Such examples are endless as the endless possibilities we encounter in our daily or professional lives.

One may therefore equate our lives to an on-going apprenticeship. In early childhood, under the watchful eyes of our parents, and later influenced by contacts with other people and continuously changing environment, we store models of behaviour for any given situation. This process goes on all the time, practically until death, because every day new situations and challenges await us, resulting in continuously increasing amount of models of behaviour stacking up in our minds. The more such models the better we are prepared to deal with new situations coming our way. In early life such "apprenticeship" is very fruitful and intense compared to older age, because children and youngsters are like sponges in absorbing information from many more sources.

Going back to Oscar's case, it is not my intention to excuse him from killing Reeva. Killing is a crime and should be punished. However, in order to deliver a just sentence one should analyze this case from many perspectives looking for mitigating factors which could even set him free.

Someone who has never killed any being, even an animal, would not know how it feels and how one would behave in such a situation. On the other hand, a serial killer may find pleasure in doing it repeatedly. This is why an explanation of Oscar's behaviour may be difficult. He has never murdered anyone before and must have been acting under severe stress during the unfortunate killing of Reeva.

One should also consider the scarcity of information concerning their private lives. We know quite a lot about Oscar's sport career but not too much about Reeva's earlier attempts to enter the world of modelling. Even the fact that Oscar and Reeva were an item, was publicized after this tragedy with a multitude of stories about their great love and/or hate which, in fact, mutually excluded one another. Mass-media published a lot of sentimental articles about her love and devotion to him, although still denied by one member of her close family, aired on a popular American TV channel, when he said: *"she did not love him"*. Similar sentiments were shared by Reeva's mother whilst disclosing a revelation about their continuous fights and quarrels.

Where is the truth? If they loved one another so much why did they spend so much of their precious time apart that night, with her apparently doing Yoga and him busy elsewhere? We don't know what they really did that night, but apparently at 3 am he woke up with a start hearing strange noises in the house, which he assumed to be a break-in.

Witnesses say that the couple was arguing violently and throughout the night. If this is true, did he demand her commitment and she refused? Did she say something which infuriated him beyond the possibility of self-restrain? Perhaps on seeing what she had done she got scared and hid away in the toilet, cell phones in her hands, locking the door behind her, which according to her ex-boyfriend Warren Lahoud was unlike her. Did she try to summon help? A few weeks earlier, when Oscar was driving too fast with her in the car, she got scared of his recklessness and phoned her mother begging her to pacify him. If this was the case, we will most probably never know why this time she couldn't stop him and why, blind with rage, he began shooting through the door.

Some published facts about Oscar's last few years may support such a possibility. At the start of his sport career everybody perceived him as a nice youngster with a boyish smile. Later, unfortunately, he began changing. Most probably it didn't happen suddenly. It had to be a continuous process, as continuous as the interaction of our brains with the environment. The most important and/or traumatizing corner stones of his life, like the amputation of his lower legs, getting new prostheses, divorce of his parents, death of his mother and later rising of his status as a celebrity had to crucially influence his mind. Finally, life in a fast track of fame and money, whilst chased by paparazzi and fuelled by populist daily press probably crown it all, convincing him of being on top of the universe. Perhaps this feeling that he could do anything he desired caused his ego to change slowly, albeit for the worse.

To make matters even more complicated one of the most important elements of his life was continuously missing: a woman. He needed one to complete his life, perhaps not only to satisfy his lust, but also as a companion and a confidante. Like his mother whom he dearly missed. This is why, while searching for the perfect partner he became *"'n rokjagter"*. (skirt chaser)

But moving around in circles of wealth and celebrities he could not find anybody closely resembling his mother. I know little about such "high" and wealthy societies, but I suppose money is god and friendships are meaningless. This is why it is more tempting for me to think of Reeva rather as a gold digger than his true love. This notion may fit in perfectly with the fact that she was in the process of "being discovered" as a model after they met rather than before.

Unfortunately, death silenced Reeva Steenkamp and she cannot defend herself. This leaves us with Oscar to explain his behaviour. Two others I think, who could also shed some light on the events of that fateful Valentine's Day in 2013, are former boyfriend Mr. Warren Lahoud and Oscar's close confidante, Mr. Justin Divaris. Mr. Lahoud spoke to tabloids several times already, but Mr. Divaris is silent like an old grave. Did he know what Reeva had expected of Oscar when he introduced her to him? Does he hold himself accountable for their short relationship and its tragic end?

In summary, while judging Oscar of wrongdoing we must not forget about Reeva's input into this affair. If she wanted to exploit him in order to get lucrative contracts in the modelling industry, something she could not get for years, she should also be found guilty, even if she paid the highest price. Criminal lawyers are familiar with cases of murders on demand: anyone who hires an assassin to kill another person must be brought to justice. Looking from that perspective Reeva must also be on trial, shoulder to shoulder with Oscar. Otherwise the judgement pronounced on him may not be fair.

To me the relationship between Reeva Steenkamp and Oscar Pistorius sounded strange right after I heard about it. If she used him for her personal gain, still maintaining close relationships with her former boyfriends, while denying Oscar full commitment and love, she most probably warranted her own death.

- ∞ -

Even before I began studying the functioning of the human brain the above scenario seemed to me the most probable. I was convinced that Reeva went into her relationship with Oscar with eyes wide open, knowing exactly what she wanted of him. I thought that it never crossed her mind that Oscar might be so psychologically unstable that stringing him along would end up with a tragedy.

She might have been prone to make such a mistake because on the surface Oscar looked a very successful and happy young man. Knowing him closely for a few months only she could not have been fully aware of the fact that everything he achieved was due to his incredible determination, perseverance and hard work against all odds, since he was 11 months old, when he got his first prosthetic limbs.

Most of us try to create "sheltered" conditions for us and our children at homes, places to play, learn and work. Only tragedies, which cause our worlds to tumble down like a house of cards, plainly expose the fragility of our existence. In such times we suddenly come to conclusions that our deeds and behaviour should have changed years earlier and that in fact we are completely different persons than we thought we were.

And this could have happened to Oscar, making him equally guilty of this tragedy. He might have thought of himself a better person than he really was not realizing that right from birth the conditions set by his parents, especially by his mother, could lead him into an inevitable tragedy. Only now, stripped off all his glory as an international sport hero and a role model for youngsters, the hard facts of his whole life are in plain view to be exploited by mass-media.

Oscar was born with a genetic fault, lack of tibia bones in both his lower legs, so they were amputated below the knees. This had to be an incredible handicap which he managed to overcome due to the relentless work of his mother, who forced him into thinking that he was not worse, perhaps even better, than the rest of the people around him. Understanding such a devotion of his mother, who only wanted the best for her child, one should however realise that her continuous persuasion could have created a feeling in his deepest innate that he was the best of all mankind. This might subconsciously have assured him of his invincibility, with all his personal needs being always put on a pedestal. From there on there could have been just one small step into a conviction that others around him were more or less worthless, so he could exploit them all for his own needs or satisfaction.

However, as difficult as it might be, one should rather give credit to Oscar and his mother instead of condemning them both. Healthy people don't realize just how painful it is walking on prosthetic limbs. Only after inspecting a stump of an amputee can the tragedy of such people be more easily understood and accepted.

I experienced this myself, many times seeing the upper part of the shin of my nephew's right leg, amputated below the knee about 15 years ago following a motorbike accident. Compressed all day long in a stiff rubber funnel of a high-tech and very expensive prosthetic limb, the whole stump looks terrible: always red, with thick, scaling, infected, painful and granulating skin, so much so that when he drives his car even for short distances, he removes the prosthesis to place the stump on the seat next to him, so it could "breath in" the fresh air. And this is just from ordinary walking on only one prosthetics. Oscar runs on two! How does he endure such a handicap?

Another possibility that should also cross our minds is this: if some genetic defects led to the underdevelopment of both of Oscar's tibia bones he may also suffer from other deviations, for instance in his limbic system which controls his emotions. Is it not possible that faults in this part of his central nervous system forced him to react the way he did?

We know now that the brain destroys all neurons left aside. Perhaps due to genetic or environmental errors substantial parts of Oscar's sub-cortical centres responsible for generation and controlling of emotions did not interconnect into a healthy neuronal structure and were later destroyed. Added to the relentless persuasion of his mother Oscar's central nervous system could have been moulded so differently that many rules governing the behaviour of "normal" people are not applicable to him at all.

One must also bear in mind that Oscar is still very young. Men of his age need female partners to love, to cherish, to be intimate. Could this be the reason for his eagerness to start a relationship with Reeva, when she exposed herself to him? Mother of one of his former girl friends accused him of being *"'n rokjagter"*. I think this was unfair. He wasn't *"'n rokjagter"*, he was just looking for a woman he wanted to spent the rest of his life with and couldn't find one. So he had to *"jag"* (hunt), on and on, still hoping for a miracle.

And this could be the most important reason of this tragedy. Oscar is a handsome and a very articulate man. Apparently he immediately stands out in a crowd. Girls like such men. They go for them like flies to honey. Dressed in an expensive suit, with his two prosthetic limbs hidden - he is drop dead gorgeous and every woman will go for him. And they did.

But... in bed all charms pop like a soap bubble. What beautiful woman would like to be intimate with a crippled man, if not for personal gain?

Oscar and Reeva were close for only a few months. They lived apart, but she visited him on the night before Valentine's Day. Why Valentine's Day? Was he deeply in love with her and wanted to ask her something, precisely on Valentine's Day? Did she refused, but in a very degrading way? Could this refusal have sent him into a rage, forcing her to seek shelter in the toilet, cell phones in her hands, dialling for help?

If this was the case he probably realised at that very instant that he was just a tool, not the lover he so deeply desired to be. He could have pictured himself a fool, a vehicle to elevate Reeva into high social circles, like all other women before her. This is why he snapped beyond possibility of calming down and in a blind and insane rage started shooting at the door sheltering her. At this very moment he could not had known what he was doing, probably not even aiming precisely. He could have seen the door as her defense, a barrier which had to be destroyed to get to her, so with his raging mind he might have perceived himself as shooting at the door, rather than at her.

- ∞ -

Such were my initial feelings. But later, while discovering the ever more convoluted intricacies of our brains I began wondering whether Oscar's original statement of a bathroom burglary was perhaps truthful. Strangely enough, endorphins' influence on the brain's activity might actually support such a claim.

Endorphins release and their physiological importance is still controversial, so assessing Oscar's behaviour through this filter might not be full proof. One thing, however, seems to be certain: Oscar was very active since he first got his prosthetic legs at the age of 11 months and later, when he was an exercise freak. Being a double-below knee amputee and a very active one, he had to experience extreme pain of the stumps, especially skin, because even the best and most expensive prostheses are not a substitute for normal, healthy legs. As natural "painkillers" released by our body endorphins could protect Oscar against extreme workout and pain. But endorphins also have very powerful side-effects.

Whatever the physiological or pathological mechanisms behind it Endorphins activity would have to have started in Oscar's early childhood, just after the amputation of both his lower legs. Thereafter, his parents' divorce and the death of his mother could have increased their production and secretion even more. The question is: could a high level of endorphins, practically all his life, have negatively influence his brain? As endorphins play an important role in the central nervous system and in developing depersonalization disorder this theory seems to be very probable.

Sufferers from **Depersonalization disorder** loose feeling of reality often perceived as dreams. They may experience panic attacks, feel not in control of their own bodies, speech and movement and be detached from their feelings and emotions. They may even loose convictions of their own identity. Such behaviour may interfere with their social and occupational functions so necessary for everyday existence. If this happened to Oscar his claims that he grabbed the revolver, went investigating and started shooting, because he heard noises in the toilet, should not be outwardly dismissed. One of his friends said that Oscar was a security freak, very quickly reacting to all happenings around him, almost instantly thinking that someone was attacking his home and his possessions. Could such behaviour result from depersonalization disorder caused by high levels of endorphins released into his central nervous system, for practically all his life?

Shooting through a closed door also supports the possibility of an accident rather than a purposeful or an in-rage execution, for at least two reasons. Firstly, people fearing an attack would unlikely go into an open confrontation. Suspecting the robber behind the door, by opening it Oscar would have exposed himself to danger. This is why there could be truth in the fact that in fear he would have shot through the closed door. Secondly, it is human nature to wallow in delight seeing a supposed offender suffering while "administering justice" with one's own hands. One could therefore argue that if it was really Oscar's intention to punish Reeva he would have rather shot her straight in the left eye, instead of firing at a closed door. Why specifically the left eye it is for the reader to guess. I have my own theory about this.

Some would argue against such conclusions asking: why did he not call on Reeva before shooting? The answer to this can be very simple, indeed. All of us often wake up with a start, still perceiving our surroundings as part of a dream. This is caused by the working of our brains, which often tend to mix those two realities. For Oscar, supposedly a sufferer from depersonalization disorder, discerning reality from dreams could have been even more difficult then for a healthy individual.

Let's suppose that Oscar and Reeva went to bed quietly as per his original deposition. Suddenly, at about 3 am, Oscar woke up with a start hearing some noises in the distance. As he lived alone, and being frightened, he probably would not even have thought about Reeva, who in the meantime, unknowingly to him, sneaked out of bed quietly and went into the bathroom, to sit in the toilet with her cell phones, perhaps to surf the net.

From there on we could argue as follows: if someone thinks there is an intruder in their home without seeing him or being physically attacked, one will instinctively freeze, trying to locate the source of the noise. Such a person stands still listening intensively, with a pounding heart. I seriously doubt that anybody would shout in such a situation. This could be dangerous.

So what could have happened to Oscar when he woke up at 3 am on that morning? He would have gotten up quietly and stopped breathing for a while trying to catch the lightest noise. Perhaps even involuntarily he would have put on his prosthetics. Eventually, on hearing taping, unusual at that time of night in his flat, he would have quietly followed the source of the noise. On hearing someone behind the closed door, and being afraid of robbers, he would have begun shooting without even thinking. And only thereafter he would have recalled that Reeva was also with him that night, and called out to her. Alas she was not in bed, where he saw her last on the previous evening. In that instant he could have realized that it was her making the noise in the toilet and that he had shot her by mistake. The fact that he had to break down the closed toilet door with a cricket bat may prove such a hypothesis.

Bearing in mind that people tend to hide their true emotion and that Oscar has now the most compelling reasons to do so, it might not be that easy to confirm such a hypothesis fully. Nobody could have predicted Reeva's untimely death at the hands of this world-renown sport hero. I don't think that Oscar has ever been tested for levels of hormones in his body. Before this tragedy he was perceived as a nice boy, so it would have been difficult to expect of him to have undergone a full psychological examination. If this is the case there is no reference point to which one could compare his state of mind while he was seemingly "normal" to one after the attack on Reeva and to draw some binding conclusions.

I think that without a proper explanation of Oscar's state of mind during shooting this case will never be closed. This may cause even more unnecessary damage, not only to Reeva's parents but also to the wellbeing of Oscar who, in my mind, no matter if acquitted or not, is already charged and sentenced for life.

Physiologically incorrect, politically correct equality

I don't know the outcome of Oscar's case. I also don't know whether the theory I presented above is correct. I have no way whatsoever to prove it. I am not a psychologist, psycho-pathologist or a researcher in the field of the altered state of mind. But if I am right, if Oscar's behavioural instability was caused by his differently formed brain, his case should raise a red flag concerning our civilization.

I am convinced that both Oscar and Reeva are typical examples of ills that bother our societies, no matter in which country and on what continent and I am very deeply concerned about it. The fact that people resort to violence, be it the most "powerful" statesmen of the world or be it home bullies, should make us all wary that the world we created for ourselves is sick to the core.

We are the civilization of killers and fast fixers. From the biological point of view man became the biggest threat to the balance of life on Earth and the most dangerous threat to his own existence who – before he hangs down in the noose he made for himself – would break all branches of the tree he is sitting on. But we think we can afford it in the name of wrongly understood human rights, financial gain, power and democracy. We kill the Earth, murdering thousand of species, some before even discovering them. We pump crude oil out of the ground causing tremendous environmental damage, and while prospecting for it we resort to powerful ground explosions which may be the reasons of tectonic shifts, earthquakes and tsunamis. We destroy the atmosphere by infesting it with enormous amounts of carbon dioxide, radioactive waste, chemicals or smog which cause climate change and threaten our health. We carry out dangerous genetic experiments, producing genetically changed species which may cause a breaking down of the delicate balance of all genetic traits set up by Mother Nature during million years of evolution. Some crazy scientists even try making completely new bacteria, to clean spilled crude oil and to produce fuel. But as scientists shouldn't they know that their bacteria may escape the confinement and threaten all organic life on Earth?

If we do all of the above, and much, much more, who are we, really, to judge Oscar and Reeva? And most of all, do we notice the deepest message of Oscar's and Reeva saga which from the logical point of view is the negation of all that supposed "humanity" has stood for since the beginning of the Renaissance?

Observing the media circus around the Oscar's case, "the case of the century" as they call it, I wonder how many people give to it much more significance than just a tragic case of a woman killed by a man. How many people realize that this case sends a very powerful message to all political, sociological, religious or judicial leaders and to all people all over the world. This message reads: we are not born equal!

There cannot be equality when all of us don't look alike. If we were, we would all be, say, the same sized, shaped and coloured cardboard boxes. There cannot be equality when some of us are bigger while others are smaller, fatter or thinner, with differently coloured eyes and hair, smooth skins or pimples. There cannot be equality when some of us live longer but some die a few days after birth due to congenital defects. There cannot be equality when we speak different tongues, worship different gods, and continually pick on whose God is different from ours, because ours is the right one. Such a list of inequalities can go on forever and yet most ordinary people are brainwashed into thinking that we are... all equal?

But most of all, there cannot be equality when our brains, these most important organs, since the very first day of fertilization slowly grow in such a probabilistic process that even now we can hardly recognize and name all crucial steps of its creation. We know that in the first three months of gestation up to 80% of our whole genome works laboriously to create and anchor billions of proto-neurons of the central nervous system. We know that later, while already in their posts these proto-neurons start growing an extremely convoluted net of connections. A net which also grows probabilistically, in complete dependence on the environment and on the set of six senses connecting them together. And to make this process even so much more complicated both brain and all senses still mature while growing, resulting after almost three decades with a fully developed human being. A being different from all 7 billion around him!

Knowing all this it is really extremely difficult to agree with an officially accepted and politically correct notion that we are all born equal.

For the roots of this notion one should look at Thomas Jefferson's "Declaration of Independence" which says: *"We hold these truths to be self-evident, that all men are created equal, that they are endowed by their Creator with certain unalienable Rights, that among these are Life, Liberty and the Pursuit of Happiness".*

It all sounds so wonderful. However, it seems that the Founding Fathers of the thirteen American colonies thought only about themselves. Why did they not envisage that the development and strengthening of the Caucasian race on the American soil would result in the terrible slaughter of the Red Indians, for almost 50 000 years the rightful owners of the New World? Why in the centuries that followed did American politicians and ordinary citizens never object to maiming Indians in the most horrific way? Why did they not stick to the notion that all men were equal? Were the Red Indians less equal? Is the creation of the United States of

America based on the most hypocritical lie and the genocide, although enshrined in the Declaration of Independence?

Professor Frank LaPena of the Native American studies wryly says: *There was a person, up in the Humboldt County, who found a small child, a young Indian child. And they ask him "What are you doing with this child?" He said "I am protecting him. He's an orphan" And they say "Well, how do you know he's orphan?" He said "I killed his parents."*

But the case does not end there. The struggle of the American colonies against British rule had been closely observed by France, which being a staunch enemy of Great Britain secretly funded them, apparently to the tune of 100 million pounds, at that time an extravagant sum. This brought France to the verge of bankruptcy resulting in the French Revolution, although not affecting the British on their Isles.

Historians still argue about the causes of the French Revolution but one thing is certain. Just like in the American Colonies the French citizens' onslaught against their authorities was carried on under the banner of human justice and equality. The French "Declaration of the Rights of Man and of the Citizen", influenced by the American "Declaration of Independence" is its simple proof.

But there is a catch in the beautiful phrases of both of these documents. As much as the American Founding Fathers didn't need to worry about their savage Red Indians, whom they anyway considered less than animals, the revolted French knew they had a problem in their hands. At that time only about $1/7^{th}$ of the French population could obtain full political rights under their Declaration. That's why the Jacobins introduced a concept of an Active and Passive citizen, in this astute way excluding the great majority of their people from political activity.

And this simple move by the revolutionized French authority cannot be seen other than an admission of the hopelessness of this problem. Although they did not know the science of brain creation at that time the Jacobins were still aware that their Declaration was just a collection of beautiful words, impossible to implement.

Now, however, I believe that our present knowledge about the development of the human brain, unknown to Founding Fathers on both sides of the Atlantic Ocean, can set the case straight. Human equality is just one of the myths used by clever paid politicians to further their own aspirations of becoming leaders. In this way they can get into the inner circle of individuals presented with enormous powers and riches. In this way they become the *Demos* (Greek word for People), which ordinary *Plebeians* will never be.

I think that Oscar's life was full of tragedies, which he overcame due to relentless efforts by his mother and himself. This created him the way he is, different from most others, strong and arrogant. One can like it or not but one must accept that his brain is built differently, so he acts differently, therefore he cannot be measured with the same set of rules as others.

Looking from this point of view Oscar's trial is just logical nonsense. If this is the case one either has to set up a new set of rules, applicable only to him as a unique person or set him free, because the existing ones do not apply to him. This in fact is not a joke as it has happened already in the past. Apparently clever judges at the Nuremberg trial did precisely that. Expecting that Germany's war criminals would defend themselves by claiming that they followed Hitler's orders they secretly removed such paragraphs from the Allies military code books and armed in this way they could sentence the German leaders within their own discretion, many of them to death.

Looking from the similar perspective it seems the penitentiary system with its parole and probation is probably a big failure. Many English philosophers, like John Howard and Jonas Hanway thought that penal solitude could help criminals recover spiritually. Solitude was supposed to be a place to repent one's sins. How could they know however, that this was just wishful thinking? How could they know that the creation of the human brain depends far more on the environment than on the genetic make up? How could they know that once this process is completed it could not be reversed in any way?

This probably is true considering that all proto-neurons of the growing brain of the foetus are in their right places already at the end of the third month of gestation. Thereafter, for the next six months they make interconnections in the process which continues for the next two years after birth. Myelination of some axons may take up to almost three decades. These all clearly indicate the complexity and length of the brain's creation.

Complexity of behaviour and the morality of inmates are very well portrayed in a film "Straight Time". Here Dustin Hoffman plays the role of a parolee, who in the end returns to his old criminal ways. Although he is pushed to it by a parole officer, nevertheless it is his way of life because he has known no other since he was a child. His brain, influenced by the environment he was born into and grew up in conditioned him to do what he was doing the best: stealing. I think that makers of this film, probably unintentionally, made a statement that the brains of the most hardened criminals will never allow them to return to the path of straight citizens. Their brains were created in a very specific way and nothing could change it.

Epilogue

Since a few words about Einstein's the Principle of Relativity opened this text it is probably right to close it in a similar fashion. I think that the Theory of Relativity has a direct bearing on Oscar's case by correlating very closely with the working of the human mind. If the most brilliant brains can come up with striking theories like the Big Bang or Branes and the theory of a Cyclic Ekpyrotic Universe, how much damage could they do, should they be distorted by pathologies affecting them from early childhood? Oscar's case might be this best example.

Since I can remember I was always interested in science and technology, physics being one of my favoured subjects. I read a lot although many concepts are difficult for me to comprehend due to a variety of convoluted mathematical equations which, somehow, I cannot picture properly in my inferior frontal lobes. This is why I admire scientists a lot, one of them being Professor Brian Cox, whom I consider a genius. His frontal lobes must be really uniquely developed allowing him lighting fast trips to far away boundaries of our Universe and equally fast comebacks, arriving younger each time.

Physicists say that our Universe was created about 14 billion years ago by an event called the Big Bang, when somewhere and suddenly an infinitely small, hot and explosive singularity came into being out of the blue (as far as I understand nobody knows yet what that "blue" was) and exploded violently giving rise to space/light/time reality. This, by further expansion and cooling matured and coalesced into galaxies, stars and planets of the Universe that we know today.

Theories concerning the beginning of the Universe fill volumes of popular science books, more often then not difficult to grasp especially if they are speckled with formulae understandable only to scientists. The Queen of Sciences, Mathematics, seems to be malleable in their hands so it is difficult to argue with these gentlemen who every day oppress the keyboards of their computers furiously and fly on the shoulders of neutrinos on long trips somewhere into the unknown, otherwise not accessible to normal folk.

However, many years ago in one of the textbooks on mathematics I found a very convoluted yet doubtless proof that $2 + 2 = 5$. Taking this as an example, I suppose clever mathematics can prove anything, so I would like to ask physicists a few questions.

If just in a split of a second before the Big Bang, there was a singularity of whatever characteristic and origin, it must have been building up for a considerably long period beforehand, similar to the yearly genesis of hurricane-bearing singularities in the belt of the Atlantic Ocean just north of the equator. Such a singularity had to be suspended somewhere, in a medium or in space or in something else, of whatever characteristic and origin. If this is the case the three-dimensional co-ordinates of such a singularity suspended who-knows-where and by who-knows-what, (or Who?) had to be well defined. This implies that 3D measurements of distances had to define such co-ordinates as well. One therefore cannot resist the conclusion that distances/measurements/space had to exist well before the Big Bang. It follows that one should treat them as separate, much earlier entities, so to say Before-Big-Bang entities (BBB), unlike light/time entities, created After Big Bang (ABB). The overall conclusion of such an interpretation is this: light and time came into being after the Big Bang, so they both can't be mixed with the space and distance which should have existed well before the Big Bang, even if this existence defies mathematical description.

To support such thinking let's imagine the following: scientists are certain about the existence of Black Holes even though the Event Horizon prevents them from being seen. And yet they do describe their characteristics mathematically. By parallel, can't they calculate back 14 billion years of the Universe's existence, pass-by the "event horizon" of the Big Bang and with mathematical formulae "see" what was there before? Perhaps by doing so one would be able to get to the origin of the Pan-Universal XYZ Co-Ordinates of the Big Bang's singularity, allowing us to use it as a point of reference for momentum of all galaxies and stars of our Universe? This would support Newton rather than Einstein. It could also be comparable to one of the milestones of algebra, i.e. invention of the "Zero" by Aryabhata. Assuming the Big Bang's singularity just as a single point, but not Beginning of only our own Universe, on the 3D graph of the Pan-Universe's perpetual existence, and perhaps denoting it with an infinity sign, could turn upside down all our astrophysical concepts. It could also be the final *coup de grâce* to Einstein's thinking.

According to Brian Cox and Jeff Forshaw's book "Why does $E=mc^2$?" (ISBN 978-0-306-81876-9, page 42) Albert Einstein carried out an *"often favoured thought experiment"*. Even more so, as I read a long time ago, whilst contemplating the Theory of Relativity, Einstein apparently even pictured himself flying on a ray of the Sun with the speed of light.

Who can prove anything with such thoughts? Our present knowledge about functioning of the human brain makes Einstein's *"thought experiments"* dubious right from the outset. One can think out anything, even the most fantastic ideas like walking on the surface of the Sun and in order not to grill one's feet use huge freezing boots made of liquid helium produced on site from the Sun's abundant helium and energy. The brain can do this with ease, filling gaps of our innate in a split of a second. Does it mean though, that all we can pan out in our brains is true or may one day materialize? I don't think so. But for the sake of an argument let's accept the validity of Einstein's thinking.

So what was this thought experiment of Einstein?

In short, he proposed that for a man sitting with a light clock on board a speeding train, being observed by a stationary man on the platform, the time runs slower. Einstein came to such a conclusion after designing in his own mind a light clock consisting of a one meter long stick with a light emitter and detector on its one end, and a mirror on another.

In Einstein's thought experiment the man on the train was supposed to see light, ticking exactly vertically from emitter, via mirror, back to detector. But for the man on the platform, observing the clock on the train speeding past him, this view had to be distorted due to the train's movement, the faster the train the more "opening" of the light beam at the bottom of the light clock. This opening, calculated with the Pythagorean Theorem, with the assumption of the constant speed of light of about 300 000 km/sec, would make the time run slower for the man on the train, as seen by the observer on the platform.

But now the following questions come to mind:

- Why are we so sure that a vertical movement of photons in this thought experiment will be at all visible to both men looking perpendicularly at them? A simple experiment with a flashlight can prove it wrong.

- According to Einstein it does not matter who is in motion and who is stationary, as there are no coordinates to which one can refer their movement. Suppose then, we arm both the stationary and the speedy train man with similar light clocks and let them watch one another. Obviously, both men will have to notice exactly the same lengthening of time. Could we then say that for both men the time runs equally slower, as seen by both counterparts? Should both of them age in unison? How to explain such a paradox?
- What if both men sit on the Sun's rays flying in opposite directions, observing analogous light clocks the other one grasps in their hands? How would both of them age?
- Supposing the measurements/space are BBB entities from an earlier Universe therefore of unknown characteristics, why do we mix them with light/time of the ABB entities, which rule our present Universe? In other words why are we so sure that to calculate the stretching of time one "is allowed" to use Pythagorean Theorem at all?
- Energy cannot come from nothing so there had to be something before the Big Bang. What if that BBB Universe was built only, for instance, of neutrinos? What if due to a colossal cataclysm, all neutrinos of the BBB Universe concentrated in an infinitely small point of "a space" and rose to an infinitely hot and explosive singularity, which eventually exploded as the Big Bang, destroying that Universe and creating ours? Maybe we are the legacy of that Universe gone by, so only its remains are still embedded in ours, i.e. those elusive neutrinos which cause scientists so much trouble to grasp the ungraspable? Maybe precisely those neutrinos running in all directions with the speed of light are the reservoirs of the invisible non-measurable Dark Energy and Dark Matter which originated long before the Big Bang but still influence our Universe?

One can speculate like this *ad mortem defecatem,* but the point lies elsewhere. I do not fancy quarrelling with physicists to prove or disprove the theory of relativity. I am far out of their league, but still I don't accept the easiness at which Cox and Forshaw, following Einstein's footsteps, try to equalise and interchange the world of Big Things with the world of Extra-Small Things. Writing about the muon experiment (p. 53) which supposedly proves the malleability of time, they say: *"we must therefore conclude, because the experiment tells us so, that time is malleable. Its rate of passage varies from <u>person to person (or muon to muon)</u> depending upon how they move about"*.

I do not agree with equalizing muons to persons because this defies logic of the Macro World in which we live. Why do Cox and Forshaw simply not say that it is a very unlikely possibility to substitute humans for subatomic particles, or measure all subatomic particles of the human body to allow teleportation? Subatomic particles "live" in their own mini-world of speed of light, difficult to grasp entanglement and they have the ability to fly through any space, even across atoms composing the seemingly "emptiness" of our bodies. Besides, objects accelerated to a high speed gain a lot of energy so muons, being even heavier than electrons, at the speed of 99,94 percent of that of light must really become "loaded" with energy approaching *infinitum*. What if circling with almost the speed of light muons are positioned in such a way that the centrifugal force splices electrons and tinier neutrinos together? Is it not possible that exactly this energy makes muons live longer, but not the speed itself which supposedly stretches time?

Concerning the visual perception of the Universe by our **Innate** another interesting problem arises which still gnaws my mind, i.e. seeing. In all popular books on the theory of relativity or quantum mechanics one can often find phrases "picture this" or "what could the person see". Knowing now that our minds rather than our eyes create all our visions, all attempts to explain difficult concepts of physics by asking a reader "to see" something may sometimes lead us astray.

As an example let's think about Einstein's famous question: *"what would a light beam look like if you catch up with it?"* (from: "Quantum theory cannot hurt you", by Marcus Chown, ISBN 978-0-571-23546-9, p.89)

To answer this question Chown writes: *"say you are driving a car... and catch up with another car. What does another car look like as you come abreast of it? Obviously it appears stationary"* and further: *"in exactly the same way, if you could catch up with a light beam, it ought to appear stationary, like a series of ripples frozen on a pond"*.

According to Chown, if I understood it correctly, apparently a 16 year old Einstein was already contemplating Maxwell's equations concluding that *"A stationary electromagnetic wave is an impossibility"*.

Further, Chown writes that Einstein *"had put his finger on a paradox, or inconsistency, in the laws of physics. If you were able to catch up with a beam of light, you would see a stationary electromagnetic wave, which is impossible. Since seeing impossible, is well, impossible, you can never catch up with a light beam! In other words, the thing that is uncatchable – the thing that plays the role of infinite speed in our Universe – is light."*

For a logically thinking person some important facts are still missing while contemplating the above thought car experiment. Even though both vehicles drive at the same speed next to each other their respective drivers can't see one another as stationary at all, because cars are not flat. They are 3D structures moving not only forwards but also rolling sideways with their whole bodies, twisting and turning or even sending waves of vibrations generated by the very movement of the body parts, a motor or other moving mechanisms. This, I think, could be quickly confirmed with holographic tests.

Now, let's think what could happen if we demolish both cars, piece by piece, whilst still in motion. At first we take away the top, then sides, front and back of the body, and so on and on, with the cars still running alongside each other. Eventually we get to the single atoms, still in forward motion, parallel to one another. Should they appear stationary to one another? I don't think so. Their electrons, rushing around the nuclei in different directions will preclude this. It seems that even photons, with their spins no matter in which direction, could never "see" each other as stationary, while speeding alongside one another.

Applying the above logic to the electromagnetic waves one should imagine them rather as a 3D series of rings of electrical and magnetic fields running alternately and perpendicularly to one another, stimulating and damping one another at the same time. I think that the best approximation of how such waves should "look like" is an anchor chain of the ship. A wave like this, observed from the side, could never "look" *"like a series of ripples frozen on a pond"* because from this perspective one would not be able to notice in 3D all the cross-sections of the electrical or magnetic rings, i.e. one would miss them oscillating towards and away from the observer. It seems therefore that Chown's *"ripples frozen on the pond"* is utter nonsense.

This shows the possibility of paradox conclusions arising from the "advices" of a 16 year old child preoccupied with his fantasies who didn't take into the account complicated visual processes and algorithms of his own mind. It could be strange though, to hold him accountable for this small ignorance as in-depth knowledge of the human innate did not exist in his heydays.

When I was a youngster I was also fascinated with science-fiction stories. Time travel and aging of man on Earth, while his sibling – an astronaut – was aging slower on his way through space, was a very popular subject in those days, so once I asked my father, a civil engineer: "daddy, please explain to me the theory of relativity". He looked at me, not for too long though, and with a funny grin replied: "if a man sticks his finger into another's *cytopyge* it is relative to say which one of them will be pleased".

After this answer we never returned to the topic of the theory of relativity again.

Obviously, my father used much more appropriate but cruder word than *cytopyge* (protozoa's defecating organ) not a biologist he didn't even know such a word existed. He also knew zilch about the theory of relativity and I should have expected such an answer, as by nature all his life my father was a great joker.

Nevertheless this joke fell deep into my innate and I still remember it very well. Now, so many years later and after my father's death, following 90 years of his lucky life, lucky because during WW2 he survived the Soviet's Gulag Archipelago, place where *"заключённые"* (prisoners) were expected to die in pain and sorrow, I think that his saying summarised the fact that Einstein's thinking still remains a theory, indicating that it might not be that kosher after all.

Einstein is popularly regarded as a genius. If he really was one, I rather think it's because he managed to stick his finger so deep into the physicists' *cytopyge*s and for so long that even up to this day they are unable to pull it out.

This conclusion of the Theory of Relativity I dedicate to Professor Brian Cox and all physicists hoping that while reading it they will boil up with anger and explode like a singularity of the Big Bang. I just hope though, that this will not result in the creation of many unnecessary parallel Universes in accordance with the ideas they love to promote so intensely.

- ∞ -

March – September 2013
Cape Town
South Africa

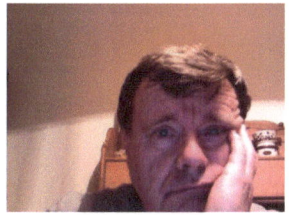

abstrzem@gmail.com

www.ingramcontent.com/pod-product-compliance
Lightning Source LLC
Chambersburg PA
CBHW040827180526
45159CB00001B/99